DBT® SKILLS TRAINING HANDOUTS AND WORKSHEETS

Also from Marsha M. Linehan

For more information and for DBT skills updates from the author,
see her websites:
www.linehaninstitute.org, http://blogs.uw.edu/brtc,
and *http://faculty.washington.edu/linehan/*

DBT® Skills Training Handouts and Worksheets

SECOND EDITION

Marsha M. Linehan

THE GUILFORD PRESS
New York   London

© 2015 Marsha M. Linehan

Published by The Guilford Press
A Division of Guilford Publications, Inc.
72 Spring Street, New York, NY 10012
www.guilford.com

Printed in the United States of America

This book is printed on acid-free paper.

Last digit is print number: 9 8 7 6 5 4 3 2 1

The author has checked with sources believed to be reliable in her efforts to provide
information that is complete and generally in accord with the standards of practice that are
accepted at the time of publication. However, in view of the possibility of human error or
changes in behavioral, mental health, or medical sciences, neither the author, nor the editor
and publisher, nor any other party who has been involved in the preparation or publication
of this work warrants that the information contained herein is in every respect accurate or
complete, and they are not responsible for any errors or omissions or the results obtained from
the use of such information. Readers are encouraged to confirm the information contained in
this book with other sources.

Library of Congress Cataloging-in-Publication Data

Linehan, Marsha.
    DBT skills training handouts and worksheets / Marsha M. Linehan. — Second edition.
       pages   cm
    Includes bibliographical references and index.
    ISBN 978-1-57230-781-0 (paperback)
    1. Dialectical behavior therapy—Problems, exercises, etc.   I. Title.
    RC489.B4L56 2015
    616.89'1420076—dc23

                             2014026331

DBT is a registered trademark of Marsha M. Linehan.

When I am on retreats, each afternoon I walk and wring my hands, saying to all the mental health patients of the world, "You don't have to wring your hands today. I am doing it for you." Often when I dance in the hallway of my house or with groups, I invite all the mental health patients of the world to come dance with me.

This book is dedicated to all the patients of the world who think that no one is thinking of them. I considered telling you that I would practice skills for you so you don't have to practice them. But then I realized that if I did, you would not learn how to be skillful yourself. So, instead, I wish you skillful means, and I wish that you find these skills useful.

About the Author

Marsha M. Linehan, PhD, ABPP, is the developer of Dialectical Behavior Therapy (DBT) and Professor of Psychology and of Psychiatry and Behavioral Sciences and Director of the Behavioral Research and Therapy Clinics at the University of Washington. Her primary research interest is in the development and evaluation of evidence-based treatments for populations with high suicide risk and multiple, severe mental disorders.

Dr. Linehan's contributions to suicide research and clinical psychology research have been recognized with numerous awards, including the Gold Medal Award for Life Achievement in the Application of Psychology from the American Psychological Foundation and the James McKeen Cattell Award from the Association for Psychological Science. In her honor, the American Association of Suicidology created the Marsha Linehan Award for Outstanding Research in the Treatment of Suicidal Behavior.

She is a Zen master and teaches mindfulness and contemplative practices via workshops and retreats for health care providers.

Preface

Since the publication of the original Dialectical Behavior Therapy (DBT) skills training manual in 1993, there has been an explosion of research on the applications of DBT across disorders. My pilot and first DBT study focused on the treatment of highly suicidal adults. Now, we have research demonstrating the efficacy of DBT skills training with suicidal adolescents, as well as adults with borderline personality disorder, eating disorders, treatment-resistant depression, substance use, and a variety of other disorders. A diagnosis of a mental disorder is not required, however, to benefit from DBT skills. Friends and family members of individuals with difficulties will find these skills helpful; kids in elementary school through high school can gain from these skills. Businesses will find DBT skills useful in creating better work environments. All the DBT therapists I know practice these skills in their own lives on a routine basis. I myself am grateful for the skills because they have made my life a lot easier. As someone once said to me, "Aren't these skills your mother was supposed to teach you?" I always say yes, but for many people their mother just did not or was not able to get around to it.

I developed many of the skills by reading treatment manuals and treatment literature on evidence-based behavioral interventions. I reviewed what therapists told their patients to do and then repackaged those instructions in skills handouts and worksheets and wrote teaching notes for therapists. For example, the skill "opposite action" is a set of instructions based on exposure-based treatments for anxiety disorders. The major change was to generalize the strategies to fit treatment of emotions other than anxiety. "Check the facts" is a core strategy in cognitive therapy interventions. The mindfulness skills were a product of my 19 years in Catholic schools, my training in contemplative prayer practices through the Shalem Institute's spiritual guidance program, and my 35 years as a Zen student—and now Zen master. Mindfulness of current thoughts also draws from acceptance and commitment therapy. In general, DBT skills are what behavior therapists tell clients to do across many effective treatments. Some of the skills repurpose entire treatment programs now formulated as a series of steps. The new "nightmare protocol," an emotion regulation skill, is an example of this. Other skills came from research in cognitive and social psychology. Still others came from colleagues developing new DBT skills for new populations. As you can see, these skills came from many different sources and disciplines.

I am happy to present this skills training manual for clients, which includes all of the handouts and worksheets I have developed so far in DBT. (Stay tuned for more.) You are not likely to need to use all of the skills I have included. Every skill works for someone and no skill works for everyone. The skills in this book have been tested with a huge variety of people: adults, adolescents, parents, friends, and families, both high risk and low. I hope the skills are just what you need. Use your interpersonal skills (see the DEAR MAN GIVE FAST skills in the Interpersonal Effectiveness skills module) to talk your skills trainer or other teacher into teaching you skills not ordinarily covered in skills training if you want to learn them. If you should decide to venture forth on your own, I must tell you that we have no research on the effectiveness of this skills manual as a self-help workbook or self-treatment manual. I am hoping to write a self-help treatment book in the future, so keep your eyes open for that. Meanwhile, you might be interested in the skills videos available through The Guilford Press or The Linehan Institute and listed on page ii of this manual. They themselves do not constitute treatment, but we know that many people have nonetheless found them useful, even though we have not collected data on them. On your own or with the help of a skills teacher, I wish you skillful means.

Acknowledgments

Developing, researching, testing, and organizing the behavioral skills in this book has been a process that has unfolded over many years. Over these years many people made important contributions to what finally became this set of skills and worksheets. Here I want to thank a long line of teachers, colleagues, students, postdoctoral fellows, and clients, who for many years have been in dialogue with me on how to best develop, organize, explain, and disseminate behavioral skills to those in need of skillful means.

I want to acknowledge Rev. Pat Hawk and Rev. Willigis Yaeger, who were my contemplative prayer and Zen teachers, and Anselm Romb, my Franciscan spiritual guide, who taught me to let go of words. Each of them listened to me for hours as I sorted out how to practice and how to teach mindfulness. My mentors, Gerald Davison and Marvin Goldfried, taught me behavior therapy, and through them I was introduced to evidence-based treatments, where I found most of the skillful means that I condensed into the skills in this book. I extend my gratitude to Jon Kabat-Zinn, John Teasdale, Mark Williams, and Zindel Segal for inspiration. I especially want to thank my students and former students (in alphabetical order), Milton Brown, Anita Lungu, Andrada Neacsiu, Shireen Rizvi, Stephanie Thompson, Chelsey Wilks, Brianna Woods; and my fellows and former fellows, Alex Chapman, Eunice Chen, Melanie Harned, Erin Miga, Marivi Navarro, and Nick Salsman. Many others have jumped in when asked, colleagues Seth Axelrod, Kate Comtois and her entire DBT team, Sona Dimidjian, Anthony Dubose, Thomas Lynch, and Suzanne Witterholt, as well as the Linehan Institute scientific advisory committee (Martin Bohus, Alan Fruzzetti, André Ivanoff, Kathryn Korslund, and Shelley McMain). I could not have written this book without the help of Elaine Franks, my fabulous administrative assistant, and Thao Truong, our office and financial manager, who made sure that our research clinic did not fall apart while everyone was waiting for me to finish this book. My family, Geraldine, Nate, Catalina, and Aline, made life easy at every turn no matter the stress—not a minor contribution to getting a book written.

Much of what is in this manual I learned from the many clients who participated in skills training groups that I have conducted over the years. I am grateful to all those who put up with the many versions that did not work or were not useful, and to those among them who gave enough feedback for me to make needed revisions in the skills being taught.

The clients who gave feedback were, for the most part, individuals at high risk for suicide. I thank the University of Washington Human Subjects Division, which has never even once impeded my research treating individuals at extremely high risk for suicide. Their willingness to allow such high-risk research when other universities often do not sets an example and made this book possible.

Last, but certainly not least, I want to thank my copy editor, Marie Sprayberry, Senior Editor Barbara Watkins, Executive Editor Kathyrn Moore, and the staff at The Guilford Press. In getting this manual out in a timely fashion they each had occasion to practice all the distress tolerance skills in this book. Their concern for this book and for this form of treatment was evident at every step.

Alas, it is likely that I have forgotten or accidently left out one or more individuals who have contributed to this book. If so, please let me know so I can include you in future editions.

Contents

Mindfulness Skills

Mindfulness Handouts

Mindfulness Worksheets

Worksheets for Core Mindfulness Skills

Worksheets for Other Perspectives on Mindfulness Skills

Interpersonal Effectiveness Skills

Interpersonal Effectiveness Handouts

Worksheets for Building Relationships and Ending Destructive Ones

Worksheets for Walking the Middle Path

Emotion Regulation Skills

Emotion Regulation Handouts

Handouts for Understanding and Naming Emotions

Handouts for Changing Emotional Responses

Handouts for Reducing Vulnerability to Emotion Mind

Distress Tolerance Skills

Handouts for Reality Acceptance Skills

Handouts for Skills When the Crisis Is Addiction

Distress Tolerance Worksheets

Worksheets for Crisis Survival Skills

Purchasers can download and print the worksheets
from this book at *www.guilford.com/dbt-worksheets*.

Introduction to This Book

This book contains informational handouts and worksheets for people learning Dialectical Behavior Therapy (DBT) skills. The overall goal of DBT skills training is to help you increase your resilience and build a life experienced as worth living. DBT skills are aimed at teaching a synthesis of how to change what is and how to accept what is. Skills teach you both how to change unwanted behaviors, emotions, thoughts, and events in your life that cause you misery and distress as well as how to live in the moment, accepting what is. There are different sets of DBT skills, and no single training program will include all of the handouts and worksheets in this book. Your skills trainer or individual therapist/case manager will direct you to the appropriate handouts and worksheets for your particular program.

How This Book Is Organized

There are five main sections in this book, and each begins with a brief introduction. Following a first section on General Skills, there is a section of handouts and worksheets for each of the four main DBT skills modules: Mindfulness Skills, Interpersonal Effectiveness Skills, Emotion Regulation Skills, and Distress Tolerance Skills. There are topical subsections of handouts and worksheets within each skills module, as described below. Every skill or set of skills has a corresponding handout with instructions for practicing that skill. Nearly every handout has at least one (often more than one) associated worksheet for recording your practice of the skill. The introductions to each section summarize the handouts, their purposes, and the worksheets that go with them.

General Skills: Orientation and Analyzing Behavior

During **Orientation**, you will be introduced to DBT and the goals of skills training, and will be encouraged to identify your own personal goals. You will also be oriented to the format, rules, and meeting times of your particular skills program.

The handouts and worksheets for this portion of General Skills cover skills training goals, guidelines, assumptions, and DBT's biosocial theory. Biosocial theory is an explanation of why some people find it challenging to manage their emotions and actions. Also included in this section are handouts and worksheets for two skills for **Analyzing Behavior**: chain analysis and missing-links analysis. These skills are often taught in individual DBT, but they may also be taught at any point during skills training.

Mindfulness Skills

Following a brief presentation on **Goals and Definitions**, the handouts and worksheets for the Mindfulness module focus on **Core Mindfulness Skills**. These skills are central in DBT: They teach how to observe and experience reality as it is, to be less judgmental, and to live in the moment with effectiveness. They are the first skills taught, and they support all the other DBT skills. DBT mindfulness skills are translations of meditation practices from Eastern and Western spiritual traditions into specific behaviors that you can practice. No spiritual or religious convictions are expected or necessary for practicing and mastering these skills.

Other Perspectives on Mindfulness includes several subsets of handouts and worksheets. A Spiritual Perspective (including Wise Mind from a Spiritual Perspective and Practicing Loving Kindness) is a set of handouts and worksheets included for those who consider spirituality an important part of their lives. The skills covered here focus on experiencing ultimate reality, sensing our intimate connection with the entire universe, and developing a sense of freedom. The Skillful Means: Balancing Doing Mind and Being Mind set focuses on balancing two seeming polarities: working to achieve goals, while at the same time letting go of attachment to achieving goals. The handouts and worksheets for Wise Mind: Walking the Middle Path cover skills for finding a synthesis of extremes.

Interpersonal Effectiveness Skills

The handouts and worksheets in the Interpersonal Effectiveness module help you manage interpersonal conflicts effectively and maintain and improve relationships with other people (those you are close to, as well as strangers). After a short introduction on **Goals and Factors That Interfere**, there are three main sets of these forms. The first set is focused on **Obtaining Objectives Skillfully**. These are strategies for asking for what you want, saying no to unwanted requests, and doing this in a way that maintains your self-respect and keeps others liking you. The handouts and worksheets for **Building Relationships and Ending Destructive Ones** help you find potential friends, get people to like you, maintain positive relationships with others, and (when necessary) end destructive relationships. This module's handouts and worksheets for **Walking the Middle Path** are about walking a middle path in your relationships, and balancing acceptance with change in yourself and in your relationships with others.

Emotion Regulation Skills

The handouts and worksheets in the Emotion Regulation module help you to manage your emotions, even though complete emotional control cannot be achieved. To a certain extent, we all are who we are, and emotionality is part of us; however, we can learn to have more control. There are four sets of these forms. The first set covers **Understanding and Naming Emotions.** Emotions serve important functions, and it can be hard to change an emotion if you don't understand what it does for you. The second set covers **Changing Emotional Responses.** These handouts and worksheets help you reduce the intensity of painful or unwanted emotions, such as anger, sadness, shame, and so forth. They also tell you how to change situations that cause painful or unwanted emotions. **Reducing Vulnerability to Emotion Mind** is the third set. The strategies covered here increase your emotional resilience and make you less likely to become extremely or painfully emotional. The final set of handouts and worksheets deals with **Managing Really Difficult Emotions.**

Distress Tolerance Skills

The handouts and worksheets in the Distress Tolerance module help you learn to tolerate and survive crisis situations without making things worse. There are two main sets of these forms. The **Crisis Survival Skills** set covers techniques for tolerating painful events, urges, and emotions when you cannot make things better right away. The **Reality Acceptance Skills** set shows you how to reduce suffering by helping you accept and enter fully into a life even when it is not the life you want. This module also includes a set of specialized handouts and worksheets for **When the Crisis Is Addiction.**

Numbering of Handouts and Worksheets

Within each of this book's five main sections, handouts for each module are grouped together first, followed by worksheets.

Every handout has a number; some also have a letter. The latter are supplements to handouts with the same number. For example, Mindfulness Handout 3 is the main handout for the skill of Wise Mind. Mindfulness Handout 3a is supplementary and lists ways that Wise Mind can be practiced. (Worksheets are numbered in a separate sequence, as described below.) Most, but not all, handouts have corresponding worksheets that can be used for recording skills practice. Associated worksheets are listed by number next to the handouts in the table of contents, as well on the handouts themselves.

There are multiple alternative worksheets associated with many of the handouts. There are worksheets that cover all the skills in a section, as well as worksheets that cover individual skills. For example, Mindfulness Worksheets 2, 2a, 2b, and 2c all cover the same core mindfulness skills, and so each carries the same number, 2. However, each worksheet is formatted a bit differently, and the worksheets vary as to how many practices they can accommodate. The handouts associated with worksheets are listed by number next to the worksheets in the table of contents, as well as on the worksheets themselves.

Not all DBT skills programs teach all the modules or all the skills in each module. Even those that do cover all the modules will not necessarily use every handout and worksheet. You are, however, likely to use some worksheets multiple times. For this reason, the author and publisher grant you, the book purchaser, permission to make photocopies of handouts and worksheets in this volume for your personal use. You can also download and print out copies of the worksheets from *www.guilford.com/dbt-worksheets*.

GENERAL SKILLS: ORIENTATION AND ANALYZING BEHAVIOR

Introduction to Handouts and Worksheets

There are two sets of handouts and worksheets in this part of the book. The first covers **Orientation**, which typically takes place during the first session of a new skills group, or when new members join an ongoing skills group. The purpose of orientation is to introduce members to one another and to the skills trainers, and to orient members to the format, rules, and meeting times of the particular skills training program. As described below, General Handouts 1 through 5 cover these issues, along with General Worksheet 1. General Handouts 6 through 8, and their corresponding worksheets, cover two important general skills for **Analyzing Behavior:** chain analysis and missing-links analysis. These are also described below.

Orientation

• **General Handout 1: Goals of Skills Training.** This handout lists the general and the specific goals of DBT skills training. Use this handout to think how you could personally benefit from skills training. Which areas are you most interested in? Use **General Worksheet 1: Pros and Cons of Using Skills** any time you aren't sure whether there are benefits to practicing DBT skills. Be sure to fill out the pros and cons for both the option of practicing skills and the option of not practicing.

• **General Handout 1a: Options for Solving Any Problem.** Although there are many, many things that can cause us pain, our options for responding to pain are limited. We can solve the problem that is causing the pain. We can try to feel better by changing our emotional response to the pain. Or we can accept and tolerate the problem and our response. Each of these options requires use of one or more DBT skills. The final option is to stay miserable (or make things worse) and use no skills.*

• **General Handout 3: Guidelines for Skills Training.** This handout lists the guidelines for most standard DBT skills programs. These are standards of behavior that people in a group skills program are asked to follow. Some programs may have somewhat modified guidelines.

• **General Handout 4: Skills Training Assumptions.** Assumptions are beliefs that cannot be proved. In DBT skills training, all group members and skills trainers are asked to abide by these assumptions.

• **General Handout 5: Biosocial Theory.** Biosocial theory is an explanation of how and why some people find it challenging to manage their emotions and actions. DBT skills are particularly useful for these people.

Analyzing Behavior

• **General Handout 6: Overview: Analyzing Behavior.** This handout previews the two general skills for analyzing behavior—chain analysis and missing-links analysis.

• **General Handout 7: Chain Analysis.** Any behavior can be understood as a series of linked parts. These links are "chained" together because they follow each other—one link in the chain leads to another. Chain analysis is a way of determining what has caused a behavior and what maintains it. This handout provides a series of questions (e.g., "What happened before that? What happened next?") for unlocking the links in a behavior chain that can feel stuck together. It guides you through figuring out what factors led to a problem behavior and what factors might be making it difficult to change that behavior. Knowing this is important if you want to change the behavior.

• **General Handout 7a: Chain Analysis, Step by Step.** This handout explains in greater detail how to do a chain analysis. **General Worksheet 2: Chain Analysis of Problem Behavior** is a worksheet for doing a chain analysis. Use it with General Handouts 7 and 7a, which have the same steps. **General Worksheet 2a: Example: Chain Analysis of Problem Behavior** is a completed sample version of General Worksheet 2.

• **General Handout 8: Missing-Links Analysis.** Missing-links analysis is a series of questions to help you figure out what got in the way of behaving effectively. Use it to identify why something did not happen that was needed and that you agreed to do, planned to do, or hoped to do. **General Worksheet 3: Missing-Links Analysis** can be used with this handout.

---

*This last option was suggested to me in an e-mail. Unfortunately, I simply cannot find the message so that I can properly credit the person here. Nevertheless, it was a fabulous addition.

General Handouts

Orientation Handouts

Goals of Skills Training

GENERAL GOAL

To learn how to change your own behaviors, emotions, and thoughts that are linked to problems in living and are causing misery and distress.

SPECIFIC GOALS

Behaviors to Decrease:

❑ Mindlessness; emptiness; being out of touch with self and others; judgmentalness.

❑ Interpersonal conflict and stress; loneliness.

❑ Absence of flexibility; difficulties with change.

❑ Up-and-down and extreme emotions; mood-dependent behavior; difficulties in regulating emotions.

❑ Impulsive behaviors; acting without thinking; difficulties accepting reality as it is; willfulness; addiction.

Skills to Increase:

❑ Mindfulness skills.

❑ Interpersonal effectiveness skills.

❑ Emotion regulation skills.

❑ Distress tolerance skills.

PERSONAL GOALS

Behaviors to Decrease:

1. _____

2. _____

3. _____

Skills to Increase:

1. _____

2. _____

3. _____

Options for Solving Any Problem

When life presents you with problems, what are your options?

1. **SOLVE THE PROBLEM**

   Change the situation . . . or avoid, leave, or get out of the situation for good.

2. **FEEL BETTER ABOUT THE PROBLEM**

   Change (or regulate) your emotional response to the problem.

3. **TOLERATE THE PROBLEM**

   Accept and tolerate both the problem and your response to the problem.

4. **STAY MISERABLE**

   Or possibly make it worse!

1. **TO PROBLEM-SOLVE:**

   Use interpersonal effectiveness skills

   Walking the Middle Path (from interpersonal effectiveness skills)

   Use problem-solving skills (from emotion regulation skills)

2. **TO FEEL BETTER ABOUT THE PROBLEM:**

   Use emotion regulation skills

3. **TO TOLERATE THE PROBLEM:**

   Use distress tolerance and mindfulness skills

4. **TO STAY MISERABLE:**

   Use *no* skills!

Overview:
Introduction to Skills Training

GUIDELINES FOR SKILLS TRAINING

SKILLS TRAINING ASSUMPTIONS

BIOSOCIAL THEORY
OF EMOTIONAL AND
BEHAVIORAL DYSREGULATION

Guidelines for Skills Training

1. **Participants who drop out of skills training are *not* out of skills training.**

   a. The only way out is to miss four scheduled sessions of skills training in a row.

2. **Participants who join the skills training group support each other and:**

   a. Keep names of other participants and information obtained during sessions confidential.

   b. Come to each group session on time and stay until the end.

   c. Make every effort to practice skills between sessions.

   d. Validate each other, avoid judging each other, and assume the best about each other.

   e. Give helpful, noncritical feedback when asked.

   f. Are willing to accept help from a person they ask or call for help.

3. **Participants who join the skills training group:**

   a. Call ahead of time if they are going to be late or miss a session.

4. **Participants do not tempt others to engage in problem behaviors and:**

   a. Do not come to sessions under the influence of drugs or alcohol.

   b. If drugs or alcohol have already been used, come to sessions acting and appearing clean and sober.

   c. Do not discuss, inside or outside sessions, current or past problem behaviors that could be contagious to others.

5. **Participants do not form confidential relationships with each other outside of skills training sessions and:**

   a. Do not start a sexual or a private relationship that cannot be discussed in group.

   b. Are not partners in risky behaviors, crime, or drug use.

Other guidelines for this group/notes:

_____

_____

_____

Skills Training Assumptions

**An assumption is a belief that cannot be proved,
but we agree to abide by it anyway.**

1. **People are doing the best they can.**

   All people at any given point in time are doing the best they can.

2. **People want to improve.**

   The common characteristic of all people is that they want to improve their lives and be happy.

3. **People need to do better, try harder, and be more motivated to change.***

   The fact that people are doing the best they can, and want to do even better, does not mean that these things are enough to solve the problem.

4. **People may not have caused all of our own problems, but they have to solve them anyway.****

   People have to change their own behavioral responses and alter their environment for their life to change.

5. **New behavior has to be learned in all relevant contexts.**

   New behavioral skills have to be practiced in the situations where the skills are needed, not just in the situation where the skills are first learned.

6. **All behaviors (actions, thoughts, emotions) are caused.**

   There is always a cause or set of causes for our actions, thoughts, and emotions, even if we do not know what the causes are.

7. **Figuring out and changing the causes of behavior work better than judging and blaming.**

   Judging and blaming are easier, but if we want to create change in the world, we have to change the chains of events that cause unwanted behaviors and events.

---

*But trying harder and being more motivated may not be needed if progress is steady and at a realistic rate of improvement.

**Parents and caregivers must assist children in this task.

Biosocial Theory

Why do I have so much trouble controlling my emotions and my actions?

**Emotional vulnerability is BIOLOGICAL:
It's simply how some people are born.**

❑ They are more *sensitive* to emotional stimuli; they can detect subtle emotional information in the environment that others don't even notice.

    ❑ They experience emotions *much more often* than others.

    ❑ Their emotions seem to hit for no reason, from *out of the blue.*

❑ They have more *intense* emotions.

    ❑ Their emotions hit like a *ton of bricks*.

    ❑ And their emotions are *long-lasting*.

**Impulsivity also has a BIOLOGICAL basis:
Regulating action is harder for some than for others.**

❑ They find it *very hard to restrain* impulsive behaviors.

    ❑ Often, without thinking, they do things that *get them in trouble.*

    ❑ Sometimes their *behavior seems to come out of nowhere.*

❑ They find it very *hard to be effective*.

    ❑ Their moods get in the way of *organizing* to achieve their goals.

    ❑ They *cannot control* behaviors linked to their moods.

(*continued on next page*)

An invalidating SOCIAL environment can make it very hard to regulate emotions.

❑ An invalidating environment doesn't seem to understand your emotions.
   ❑ It tells you your emotions are *invalid, weird, wrong,* or *bad*.
   ❑ It often *ignores* your emotional reactions and does nothing to help you.
   ❑ It may say things like *"Don't be such a baby!" "Quit your blubbering." "Quit being such a chicken and just solve the problem."* or *"Normal people don't get this frustrated."*

❑ People who invalidate are **OFTEN DOING THE BEST THEY CAN**.
   ❑ They *may not know* how to validate or how important it is to validate, or they *may be afraid* that if they validate your emotions, you will get more emotional, not less.
   ❑ They *may be under high stress* or time pressure, or they may have too few resources themselves.
   ❑ There may be just a *poor fit* between you and your social environment: **You may be a tulip in a rose garden.**

An ineffective SOCIAL environment is a big problem when you want to learn to regulate emotions and actions.

❑ Your environment may *reinforce out-of-control emotions and actions.*
   ❑ If people give in when you get out of control, it will be hard for you to get in control.
   ❑ If others command you to change, but don't coach you on how to do this, it will be hard to keep on trying to change.

It's the TRANSACTIONS that count between the person and the social environment.

❑ Biology and the social environment influence the person.

❑ The person reciprocates and influences his or her social environment.

❑ The social environment reciprocates and influences the person.

❑ And so on and on and on.

Handouts for Analyzing Behavior

Overview:
Analyzing Behavior

**To figure out its causes
and plan for problem solving.**

**Chain Analysis
is for when you engage in ineffective behavior.**

A chain analysis examines the chain of events that leads to
ineffective behaviors, as well as the consequences of those
behaviors that may be making it hard to change them. It also
helps you figure out how to repair the damage.

**Missing-Links Analysis
is for when you fail to engage in effective behaviors.**

A missing-links analysis helps you identify what got in the way of
doing things you needed or hoped to do, things you agreed to do,
or things others expected you to do. It also helps you problem-
solve for the future.

Chain Analysis

TO UNDERSTAND BEHAVIOR, DO A CHAIN ANALYSIS.

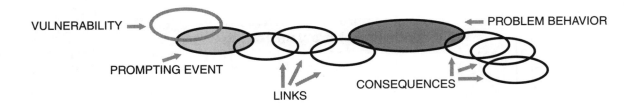

Step 1: Describe the **PROBLEM BEHAVIOR.**

Step 2: Describe the **PROMPTING EVENT** that started the chain of events leading to the problem behavior.

Step 3: Describe the factors happening before the event that made you **VULNERABLE** to starting down the chain of events toward the problem behavior.

Step 4: Describe in excruciating detail the **CHAIN OF EVENTS** that led to the problem behavior.

Step 5: Describe the **CONSEQUENCES** of the problem behavior.

To change behavior:

Step 6: Describe **SKILLFUL** behaviors to replace problem links in the chain of events.

Step 7: Develop **PREVENTION PLANS** to reduce vulnerability to stressful events.

Step 8: REPAIR important or significant consequences of the problem behavior.

Chain Analysis, Step by Step

1. **Describe the specific PROBLEM BEHAVIOR** (overeating or overdrinking, yelling at your kids, throwing a chair, having an overwhelming emotional outburst, dissociating, not coming or coming late to skills training, putting off or refusing to do skills practice, etc.).

   A. Be very specific and detailed. No vague terms.

   B. Identify exactly what *you did, said, thought, or felt* (if feelings are the targeted problem behavior). Identify what *you did not do.*

   C. Describe the intensity of the behavior and other characteristics of the behavior that are important.

   D. Describe the problem behavior in enough detail that an actor in a play or movie could recreate the behavior exactly.

   E. If the behavior is something *you did not do,* ask yourself whether (a) you did not know you needed to do it (it did not get into short-term memory); (b) you forgot it and later it never came into your mind to do it (it did not get into long-term memory); (c) you put it off when you did think of it; (d) you refused to do it when you thought of it; or (e) you were willful and rejected doing it, or some other behavior, thoughts, or emotions interfered with doing it. If (a) or (b) is the case, skip from here to Step 6 below (working on solutions). Otherwise, keep going from here.

2. **Describe the specific PROMPTING EVENT** that started the whole chain of behavior. Begin with the environmental event that started the chain. Always begin with some event in your environment, even if it doesn't seem to you that the environmental event "caused" the problem behavior. Otherwise, we could ask about any behavior, thought, feeling, or experience, "What prompted that?" Possible questions to help you get at this are:

   A. What exact event precipitated the start of the chain reaction?

   B. When did the sequence of events that led to the problem behavior begin? When did the problem start?

   C. What was going on right before the thought of or impulse for the problem behavior occurred?

   D. What were you doing/thinking/feeling/imagining at that time?

   E. Why did the problem behavior happen on that day instead of the day before?

3. **Describe specific VULNERABILITY FACTORS** happening before the prompting event. What factors or events made you more vulnerable to reacting to the prompting event with a problematic chain? Areas to examine are:

   A. Physical illness; unbalanced eating or sleeping; injury.

   B. Use of drugs or alcohol; misuse of prescription drugs.

   C. Stressful events in the environment (either positive or negative).

   D. Intense emotions, such as sadness, anger, fear, loneliness.

   E. Previous behaviors of your own that you found stressful coming into your mind.

*(**continued on next page**)*

4. **Describe in excruciating detail the CHAIN OF EVENTS** that led to the problem behavior. Imagine that your problem behavior is chained to the precipitating event in the environment. How long is the chain? Where does it go? What are the links? Write out all **links** in the chain of events, no matter how small. Be very specific, as if you are writing a script for a play. Links in the chain can be:

   A. Actions or things you do.

   B. Body sensations or feelings.

   C. Cognitions (i.e., beliefs, expectations, or thoughts).

   D. Events in the environment or things others do.

   E. Feelings and emotions that you experience.

   What exact thought (or belief), feeling, or action followed the prompting event? What thought, feeling, or action followed that? What next? What next? And so forth.

   - Look at each link in the chain after you write it. Was there another thought, feeling, or action that could have occurred? Could someone else have thought, felt, or acted differently at that point? If so, explain how that specific thought, feeling, or action came to be.

   - For each link in the chain, ask whether there is a smaller link you could describe.

5. **Describe the CONSEQUENCES** of this behavior. Be specific. (How did other people react immediately and later? How did you feel immediately following the behavior? Later? What effect did the behavior have on you and your environment?)

6. **Describe in detail** at each point where you could have used a *skillful* behavior to head off the problem behavior. What key links were most important in leading to the problem behavior? (In other words, if you had eliminated these behaviors, the problem behavior probably would not have happened.)

   A. Go back to the chain of behaviors following the prompting event. Circle each link where, if you had done something different, you would have avoided the problem behavior.

   B. What could you have done differently at each link in the chain of events to avoid the problem behavior? What coping behaviors or skillful behaviors could you have used?

7. **Describe in detail a PREVENTION STRATEGY** for how you could have kept the chain from starting by reducing your vulnerability to the chain.

8. **Describe what you are going to do to REPAIR** important or significant consequences of the problem behavior.

   A. Analyze: What did you really harm? What was the negative consequence you can repair?

   B. Look at the harm or distress you actually caused others, and the harm or distress you caused yourself. Repair what you damaged. (Don't bring flowers to repair a window you broke: fix the window! Repair a betrayal of trust by being very trustworthy long enough to fit the betrayal, rather than trying to fix it with love letters and constant apologies. Repair failure by succeeding, not by berating yourself.)

Missing-Links Analysis

**Ask the following questions to understand how and why
effective behavior that is needed or expected did not occur.**

1. **Did you know what effective behavior was needed or expected (what skills homework was given, what skills to use, etc.)?**

   IF NO to Question 1, ask what got in the way of knowing what was needed or expected. Ideas might include not paying attention, unclear instructions, never getting the instructions in the first place, becoming too overwhelmed and couldn't process the information, and so on.

   > **PROBLEM-SOLVE** what got in the way. For example, you might work on paying attention, ask for clarification when you don't understand instructions, call others, look up information, and so on.

2. **IF YES to Question 1, ask were you willing to do the needed or expected effective behavior?**

   IF NO to Question 2, ask what got in the way of willingness to do effective behaviors. Ideas might include willfulness, feeling inadequate, or feeling demoralized.

   > **PROBLEM-SOLVE** what got in the way of willingness. For example, you might practice radical acceptance, do pros and cons, practice opposite action, and so on.

3. **IF YES to Question 2, ask did the thought of doing the needed or expected effective behavior ever enter your mind?**

   IF NO to Question 3,

   > **PROBLEM-SOLVE** how to get the thought of doing effective behaviors into your mind. For example, you might put it on your calendar, set your alarm to go off, put your skills notebook next to your bed, practice coping ahead with difficult situations (see Emotion Regulation Handout 19), and so on.

4. **IF YES to Question 3, ask what got in the way of doing the needed or expected effective behavior right away?** Ideas might include putting it off, continuing to procrastinate, not being in the mood, forgetting how to do what was needed, thinking that no one would care anyway (or no one would find out), and so on.

   > **PROBLEM-SOLVE** what got in the way. For example, you might set a reward for doing what is expected, practice opposite action, do pros and cons, and so on.

General Worksheets

Orientation Worksheet

Pros and Cons of Using Skills

Due Date: _____ Name: _____ Week Starting: _____

Use this worksheet to figure out the advantages and disadvantages to you of using skills (i.e., acting skillfully) to reach your goals. The idea here is to figure out what is the most effective way for you to get what you want in life. Remember, this is about your goals, not someone else's goals.

Describe the situation or problem:
Describe your goal in this situation:

Make a list of the Pros and Cons of practicing your skills in this situation.

Make another list of the Pros and Cons for not practicing your skills or of not practicing them completely.

Check the facts to be sure that you are correct in your assessment of advantages and disadvantages.

Write on the back if you need more space.

	Practicing Skills	Not Practicing Skills
PROS	_____ _____ _____ _____	_____ _____ _____ _____
CONS	Practicing Skills _____ _____ _____ _____	Not Practicing Skills _____ _____ _____ _____

What did you decide to do in this situation? _____

_____

Is this the best decision (in Wise Mind)? _____

_____

Worksheets for Analyzing Behavior

Chain Analysis of Problem Behavior

Due Date: _____   Name: _____   Date: _____

VULNERABILITY →

PROMPTING EVENT

LINKS

CONSEQUENCES

← PROBLEM BEHAVIOR

1. What exactly is the major **PROBLEM BEHAVIOR** that I am analyzing?

2. What **PROMPTING EVENT** in the environment started me on the chain to my problem behavior? Include what happened **RIGHT BEFORE** the urge or thought came into my mind.

Day prompting event occurred: _____

3. Describe what things in myself and in my environment made me **VULNERABLE.**

Day the events making me vulnerable started: _____

(*continued on next page*)

LINKS IN THE CHAIN OF EVENTS: Behaviors (<u>A</u>ctions, <u>B</u>ody sensations, <u>C</u>ognitions/Thoughts, <u>F</u>eelings) and <u>E</u>vents (in the environment)

Possible Types of Links

A. <u>A</u>ctions

B. <u>B</u>ody sensations

C. <u>C</u>ognitions/thoughts

E. <u>E</u>vents

F. <u>F</u>eelings

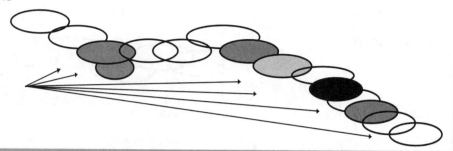

4. List the *chain of events* (specific behaviors and environmental events that actually did happen). Use the ABC-EF list above.

1st. _____

_____

2nd. _____

_____

3rd. _____

_____

4th. _____

_____

5th. _____

_____

6th. _____

_____

7th. _____

_____

8th. _____

_____

9th. _____

_____

6. List new, more *skillful* behaviors to replace ineffective behaviors. Use the ABC-EF list.

1st. _____

_____

2nd. _____

_____

3rd. _____

_____

4th. _____

_____

5th. _____

_____

6th. _____

_____

7th. _____

_____

8th. _____

_____

9th. _____

_____

(*continued on next page*)

LINKS IN THE CHAIN OF EVENTS: Behaviors (Actions, Body sensations, Cognitions/Thoughts, Feelings) and Events (in the environment)

Possible Types of Links

A. Actions

B. Body sensations

C. Cognitions/thoughts

E. Events

F. Feelings

4. List the *chain of events* (specific behaviors and environmental events that actually did happen). Use the ABC-EF list above.

10th. _____

_____

11th. _____

_____

12th. _____

_____

13th. _____

_____

14th. _____

_____

15th. _____

_____

16th. _____

_____

17th. _____

_____

6. List new, more *skillful* behaviors to replace ineffective behaviors. Use the ABC-EF list.

10th. _____

_____

11th. _____

_____

12th. _____

_____

13th. _____

_____

14th. _____

_____

15th. _____

_____

16th. _____

_____

17th. _____

_____

(*continued on next page*)

5. What exactly were the *consequences* in the environment?

And in myself?

What *harm* did my problem behavior cause?

7. *Prevention plans:*
   Ways to reduce my *vulnerability* in the future:

   Ways to prevent *precipitating event* from happening again:

8. Plans to *repair,* correct, and overcorrect the harm:

Example: Chain Analysis of Problem Behavior

Due Date: _____ Name: _____ Date: _____

Problem Behavior: _____

1. What exactly is the major **PROBLEM BEHAVIOR** that I am analyzing?

   Drinking too much and driving drunk

2. What **PROMPTING EVENT** in the environment started me on the chain to my problem behavior? Include what happened **RIGHT BEFORE** the urge or thought came into my mind.

   Day prompting event occurred: _____*Monday*_____

   My sister from out of town called me and said she was not going to come visit me the next week like she had said she would, because her husband had an important business party he wanted her to attend with him.

3. Describe what things in myself and in my environment made me **VULNERABLE.**

   Day the events making me vulnerable started: _____*Sunday*_____

   My boyfriend said he had to take a business trip sometime in the next month.

(continued on next page)

LINKS IN THE CHAIN OF EVENTS: Behaviors (<u>A</u>ctions, <u>B</u>ody sensations, <u>C</u>ognitions/Thoughts, <u>F</u>eelings) and <u>E</u>vents (in the environment)

Possible Types of Links

A. <u>A</u>ctions

B. <u>B</u>ody sensations

C. <u>C</u>ognitions/thoughts

E. <u>E</u>vents

F. <u>F</u>eelings

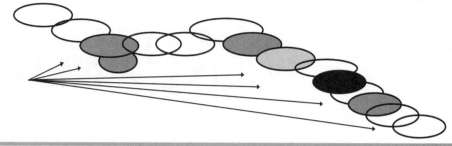

4. List the ***chain of events*** (specific behaviors and environmental events that actually did happen). Use the ABC-EF list above.

1st. *I felt hurt and started sobbing on the phone with my sister and was angry with her.*

2nd. *I thought, "I can't stand it. No one loves me."*

3rd. *I felt very ashamed once I hung up from talking to my sister.*

4th. *I thought "My life is useless; no one will ever be here for me."*

5th. *Tried watching TV, but nothing was on I liked.*

6th. *I started feeling agitated and thought, "I can't stand this."*

7th. *I decided to drink a glass of wine to feel better, but ended up drinking two whole bottles.*

8th. *Got in my car to drive to a late-night concert.*

9th. *While I was bending down to pick up a piece of paper, car swerved. I was stopped by a cop and taken in on a DUI.*

6. List new, more ***skillful*** behaviors to replace ineffective behaviors. Use the ABC-EF list.

1st. *Listen to why my sister could not come.*

2nd. *Remember that my sister and my boyfriend love me.*

3rd. *Check the facts; is my sister going to reject me over this?*

4th. *Call my sister back and apologize for being angry (since I know she will validate how I feel).*

5th. *Download a movie, work on a puzzle, or call a friend instead.*

6th. *Try my TIP skills to bring down arousal.*

7th. *Walk down the street and have a dinner out, because I won't drink too much in public.*

8th. *Call my boyfriend and ask him to come over for a while.*

9th. *Take a long bath, try TIP skills again; Keep checking the facts; remember these emotions will pass; call my therapist for help.*

(***continued on next page***)

5. **What exactly were the *consequences* in the environment?**

Short-term: I had to spend the night in jail.

Long-term: My boyfriend has less trust in me; my sister is upset about it.

And in myself?

Short-term: I am ashamed and furious with myself.

Long-term: I will have to pay more for car insurance and may have trouble getting a job.

What *harm* did my problem behavior cause?

It hurt me by giving me a DUI record. My sister feels guilty because she upset me.

7. ***Prevention plans:***

Ways to reduce my *vulnerability* in the future:

Make plans for how to cope whenever my boyfriend is out of town.

Ways to prevent *precipitating event* from happening again:

I can't keep the precipitating event from happening, so I need to practice coping ahead and have plans for how to manage when I am at home alone.

8. **Plans to *repair*, correct, and overcorrect the harm:**

Apologize to my sister and reassure her that she has a perfect right to change her plans. Work with her to plan a new time for a visit. Ask if it would be easier for her if I came to visit her.

Missing-Links Analysis

To understand missing effective behavior, do a missing-links analysis.

Due Date: _____   Name: _____   Date: _____

Missing Behavior: _____

Use this sheet to first figure out what got in the way of doing things you needed or hoped to do, or things you agreed to do or others expected you to do. Then use that information to problem-solve, so that you will be more likely to do what is needed, hoped for, or expected next time.

1. **Did I know what effective behavior was needed or expected?** Yes ____ No____

   IF NO to Question 1, what got in the way of knowing? _____

   _____

   Describe problem solving: _____

   _____ STOP

2. **IF YES** to Question 1, was I willing to do what was needed? Yes ____ No____

   IF NO to Question 2, what got in the way of wanting to do what was needed? _____

   _____

   Describe problem solving: _____

   _____ STOP

3. **IF YES** to Question 2, did the thought of doing what was needed or expected ever enter my mind? Yes ____ No____

   IF NO to Question 3, describe problem solving: _____

   _____

   _____

4. **IF YES** to Question 3, what got in the way of doing what was needed or expected right away?

   _____

   _____ STOP

   Describe problem solving: _____

   _____ STOP

MINDFULNESS SKILLS

Introduction to Handouts and Worksheets

Mindfulness is the act of consciously focusing the mind in the present moment, without judgment and without attachment to the moment. A person who is mindful is aware in and of the present moment. Mindfulness is the opposite of being on "automatic pilot," or being lost in habit. Mindfulness has to do with the quality of awareness that a person brings to everyday living. It's a way of living awake, with eyes wide open. As a set of skills, mindfulness practice is the intentional process of observing, describing, and participating in reality nonjudgmentally, in the moment, and with effectiveness (i.e., using skillful means). We can contrast mindfulness with rigidly clinging to the present moment, as if we could keep a present moment from changing if we cling hard enough. When we are mindful, we are open to the fluidity of each moment as it arises and falls away.

Goals and Definitions

  • **Mindfulness Handout 1: Goals of Mindfulness Practice.** The goals of practicing mindfulness skills, for most people, are to reduce suffering, increase happiness, and increase control of the mind. For some, a goal of mindfulness is to experience reality *as it is*. Mindfulness skills require practice, practice, practice.

  • **Mindfulness Handout 2: Mindfulness Definitions.** This handout offers basic definitions of mindfulness, mindfulness skills, and mindfulness practice.

  • **Mindfulness Worksheet 1: Pros and Cons of Practicing Mindfulness.** This worksheet is designed to help you decide whether you have anything to gain from practicing mindfulness.

Core Mindfulness Skills

The handouts and worksheets for **Core Mindfulness Skills** cover seven skills in three sets: Wise Mind; the "what" skills of observing, describing, and participating; and the "how" skills of practicing nonjudgmentally, one-mindfully, and effectively.

• **Mindfulness Worksheets 2, 2a, 2b, and 2c: Mindfulness Core Skills Practice** offer four variations for recording practice of all seven core mindfulness skills. They can be useful for recording practice after you have learned all of the core skills. **Mindfulness Worksheet 2c: Mindfulness Core Skills Calendar** offers a calendar format for recording practice of all these skills.

WISE MIND

• **Mindfulness Handout 3: Wise Mind: States of Mind.** Wise Mind is the inner wisdom that each one of us has. When we access our inner wisdom, we say we are in Wise Mind. When we enter the state of Wise Mind, we integrate opposites—including our reasonable and emotional states of mind—and we are open to experiencing reality as it is.

• You can record your practice efforts on **Mindfulness Worksheet 3: Wise Mind Practice.** (**Mindfulness Handout 3a: Ideas for Practicing Wise Mind** offers practice ideas.) Worksheet 3 asks you to rate how effective your practice was in accessing your own Wise Mind. Note that the rating is not about whether the practice calmed you or made you feel better.

MINDFULNESS "WHAT" SKILLS

• **Mindfulness Handout 4: Taking Hold of Your Mind: "What" Skills.** "What" skills are what you do when practicing mindfulness—observe, describe, or participate. Do only one of these activities at a time. To observe is to pay attention on purpose to the present moment. To describe is to put into words what you have observed. To participate is to enter into an activity fully and wholly, becoming one with whatever you are doing.

• **Mindfulness Handout 4a: Ideas for Practicing Observing, Mindfulness Handout 4b: Ideas for Practicing Describing,** and **Mindfulness Handout 4c: Ideas for Practicing Participating** offer ideas for how to practice each of the mindfulness "what" skills. If you are just learning these skills, your skills trainer is likely to assign a specific exercise or two after you first practice each skill in a session.

• **Mindfulness Worksheets 4, 4a, and 4b offer three different formats for recording practice of mindfulness "what" skills.** Worksheet 4 provides space for practice of the "what" skills only twice between sessions. **Worksheet 4a** gives space for multiple practices for each "what" skill in a checklist format. **Worksheet 4b** is aimed at those who like to write describing their practice.

MINDFULNESS "HOW" SKILLS

• **Mindfulness Handout 5: Taking Hold of Your Mind: "How" Skills.** The "how" skills are how you observe, describe, or participate—nonjudgmentally, one-mindfully, and effectively. Although the "what" skills should only be done one at a time, the "how" skills can be done together.

• **Mindfulness Handout 5a: Ideas for Practicing Nonjudgmentalness, Mindfulness Handout 5b: Ideas for Practicing One-Mindfulness,** and **Mindfulness Handout 5c: Ideas for Practicing Effectiveness** offer ideas for how to practice each of the mindfulness "how" skills. If you are just learning these skills, your skills trainer is likely to assign a specific exercise or two after you practice each one in a session.

• **Mindfulness Worksheet 5: Mindfulness "How" Skills: Nonjudgmentalness, One-Mindfulness, Effectiveness** provides space for recording only two practices of a "how" skill for the week. **Mindfulness Worksheet 5a: Nonjudgmentalness, One-Mindfulness, Effectiveness Checklist** offers a checklist format for recording "how" skills practice, and **Mindfulness Worksheet 5b: Nonjudgmentalness, One-Mindfulness, Effectiveness Calendar** offers a calendar format for this purpose. **Mindfulness Worksheet 5c: Nonjudgmentalness Calendar** is an advanced worksheet for the single skill of nonjudgmentalness.

Other Perspectives on Mindfulness Skills

There are three sets of handouts and worksheets for **mindfulness skills** that give a different perspective on mindfulness. These are Mindfulness Practice: A Spiritual Perspective; Skillful Means: Balancing Doing Mind and Being Mind; and Wise Mind: Walking the Middle Path. Some DBT skills training programs may include one or more of these sets of skills.

• **Mindfulness Handout 6: Overview: Other Perspectives on Mindfulness.** This handout briefly previews the three supplementary mindfulness skills.

MINDFULNESS PRACTICE: A SPIRITUAL PERSPECTIVE

• **Mindfulness Handout 7: Goals of Mindfulness Practice: A Spiritual Perspective.** Mindfulness can be practiced for psychological reasons or spiritual reasons. A spiritual perspective on mindfulness is included for those for whom spirituality is an important part of their life. Mindfulness practice is very old, arising initially from spiritual practices across many cultures, and it has a modern-day presence in many contemplative prayer and meditation practices.

• **Mindfulness Handout 7a: Wise Mind from a Spiritual Perspective.** This handout outlines different types of spiritual practices and includes some of the many terms used to reference the transcendent. Many spiritual and religious practices share elements in common with mindfulness practices, including silence, quieting the mind, attentiveness, inwardness, and receptivity. These are characteristics of deep spiritual experiences.

• **Mindfulness Handout 8: Practicing Loving Kindness to Increase Love and Compassion.** Anger, hate, hostility, and ill will toward ourselves and toward others can be very painful. The practice of loving kindness is a form of meditation in which specific positive words and phrases are repeatedly recited, to cultivate compassion and loving feelings as an antidote to negativity. Loving kindness is an ancient spiritual meditation practice. In some ways it is similar to praying for the welfare of ourselves and others. To record practice of loving kindness, use **Mindfulness Worksheet 6: Loving Kindness**, which provides space for describing two occasions of practicing loving kindness.

SKILLFUL MEANS: BALANCING DOING MIND AND BEING MIND

• **Mindfulness Handout 9: Skillful Means: Balancing Doing Mind and Being Mind.** "Skillful means" is a term in Zen that refers to any effective method that aids you to experience reality as it is—or, in DBT terms, to enter fully into Wise Mind. Doing mind and being mind are states of mind that, in their extreme forms, can get in the way of skillful means and of Wise Mind. Doing mind focuses on achieving goals; being mind focuses on experiencing. The polarity between them is similar to that between reasonable mind and emotion mind. In everyday life, wise living requires us to balance working to achieve goals (on the one hand), and at the very same time to let go of attachment to achieving goals (on the other hand).

• **Mindfulness Handout 9a: Ideas for Practicing Balancing Doing Mind and Being Mind.** This handout lists practice exercises. It is useful when you have already gone through mindfulness training several times.

• **Mindfulness Worksheet 7a: Mindfulness of Being and Doing Calendar, Mindfulness Worksheet 8: Mindfulness of Pleasant Events Calendar,** and **Mindfulness Worksheet 9: Mindfulness of Unpleasant Events Calendar** are all worksheets in calendar format that ask participants to record their mindfulness practice each day. The calendars focus on mindfulness during frazzled moments (Worksheet 7a), pleasant events (Worksheet 8), and unpleasant events (Worksheet 9).

WISE MIND: WALKING THE MIDDLE PATH

• **Mindfulness Handout 10: Walking the Middle Path: Finding the Synthesis between Opposites.** Wise Mind is the middle path between extremes. In Wise Mind, we replace "either–or" with "both–and" thinking in an effort to find a synthesis between oppositions. Ordinarily, when we are at an extreme on any continuum, we are in danger of distorting reality. This handout is useful if you have already gone through mindfulness training one or more times.

• **Mindfulness Worksheet 10: Walking the Middle Path to Wise Mind.** This worksheet lists several polarities that could be out of balance, and provides space for recording practice aimed at balancing them.

• **Mindfulness Worksheet 10a: Analyzing Yourself on the Middle Path.** Use this worksheet to think through whether you are out of balance on each of the polarities listed. "Out of balance" here means a living style that knocks you off your center, out of Wise Mind.

• **Mindfulness Worksheet 10b: Walking the Middle Path Calendar.** This worksheet offers opportunities for recording daily practice in a different format than in Worksheet 10. It can also be used in conjunction with Worksheet 10a.

Mindfulness Handouts

Handouts for Goals and Definitions

Goals of Mindfulness Practice

REDUCE SUFFERING AND INCREASE HAPPINESS

❑ Reduce pain, tension, and stress.

❑ Other: _____

INCREASE CONTROL OF YOUR MIND

❑ Stop letting your mind be in control of you.

❑ Other: _____

EXPERIENCE REALITY AS IT IS

❑ Live life with your eyes wide open.

❑ Experience the reality of your . . .

- connection to the universe.

- essential "goodness."

- essential validity.

❑ Other: _____

Mindfulness Definitions

WHAT IS MINDFULNESS?

- **Intentionally living with awareness in the present moment.**
  (Waking up from automatic or rote behaviors to participate and be present to our own lives.)

- **Without judging or rejecting the moment.**
  (Noticing consequences, discerning helpfulness and harmfulness—but letting go of evaluating, avoiding, suppressing, or blocking the present moment.)

- **Without attachment to the moment.**
  (Attending to the experience of each new moment, rather than ignoring the present by clinging to the past or grabbing for the future.)

WHAT ARE MINDFULNESS SKILLS?

- Mindfulness skills are the specific behaviors to practice that, when put together, make up mindfulness.

WHAT IS MINDFULNESS PRACTICE?

- **Mindfulness and mindfulness skills** can be practiced at any time, anywhere, while doing anything. Intentionally paying attention to the moment, without judging it or holding on to it, is all that is needed.

- **Meditation** is practicing mindfulness and mindfulness skills while sitting, standing, or lying quietly for a predetermined period of time. When meditating, we *focus* the mind (for example, we *focus* on body sensations, emotions, thoughts, or our breath), or we *open* the mind (paying attention to whatever comes into our awareness). There are many forms of meditation that differ mostly by whether we are opening the mind or focusing the mind—and, if focusing, depending on what is the focus of our attention.

- **Contemplative prayer** (such as Christian centering prayer, the rosary, Jewish Shema, Islamic Sufi practice, or Hindu raja yoga) is a spiritual mindfulness practice.

- **Mindfulness movement** also has many forms. Examples include yoga, martial arts (such as Qigong, tai chi, akido, and karate), and spiritual dancing. Hiking, horseback riding, and walking can also be ways to practice mindfulness.

Handouts for Core Mindfulness Skills

Overview:
Core Mindfulness Skills

WISE MIND:

STATES OF MIND

"WHAT" SKILLS

(what you do when practicing mindfulness):

Observing, Describing, Participating

"HOW" SKILLS

(how you practice when practicing mindfulness):

Nonjudgmentally, One-Mindfully, Effectively

Wise Mind:
States of Mind

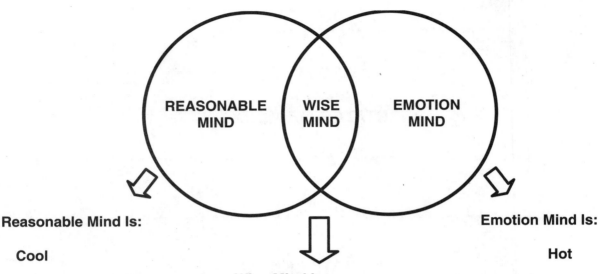

Reasonable Mind Is:

Cool

Rational

Task-Focused

When in *reasonable mind,* you are ruled by facts, reason, logic, and pragmatics. Values and feelings are not important.

Wise Mind Is:

The wisdom within each person

Seeing the value of both reason and emotion

Bringing left brain and right brain together

The middle path

Emotion Mind Is:

Hot

Mood-Dependent

Emotion-Focused

When in *emotion mind,* you are ruled by your moods, feelings, and urges to do or say things. Facts, reason, and logic are not important.

Ideas for Practicing Wise Mind

The mindfulness skills often require a *lot* of practice. As with any new skill, it is important to first practice when you don't need the skill. If you practice in easier situations, the skill will become automatic, and you will have the skill when you need it. Practice with your eyes closed and with your eyes open.

1. ❑ **Stone flake on the lake.** Imagine that you are by a clear blue lake on a beautiful sunny day. Then imagine that you are a small flake of stone, flat and light. Imagine that you have been tossed out onto the lake and are now gently, slowly, floating through the calm, clear blue water to the lake's smooth, sandy bottom.

   • Notice what you see, what you feel as you float down, perhaps in slow circles, floating toward the bottom. As you reach the bottom of the lake, settle your attention there within yourself.

   • Notice the serenity of the lake; become aware of the calmness and quiet deep within.

   • As you reach the center of your self, settle your attention there.

2. ❑ **Walking down the spiral stairs.** Imagine that within you is a spiral staircase, winding down to your very center. Starting at the top walk very slowly down the staircase, going deeper and deeper within yourself.

   • Notice the sensations. Rest by sitting on a step, or turn on lights on the way down if you wish. Do not force yourself further than you want to go. Notice the quiet. As you reach the center of your self, settle your attention there—perhaps in your gut or your abdomen.

3. ❑ **Breathing "Wise" in, "Mind" out.** Breathing in, say to yourself, "Wise"; breathing out, say "Mind."

   • Focus your entire attention on the word "wise," then, focus it again entirely on the word "mind."

   • Continue until you sense that you have settled into Wise Mind.

4. ❑ **Asking Wise Mind a question.** Breathing in, silently ask Wise Mind a question.

   • Breathing out, listen for the answer.

   • Listen, but do not give yourself the answer. Do not tell yourself the answer; listen for it.

   • Continue asking on each in-breath for some time. If no answer comes, try again another time.

(*continued on next page*)

5. ❑ **Asking is this Wise Mind?** Breathing in, ask yourself, "Is this (action, thought, plan, etc.) Wise Mind?"

   - Breathing out, listen for the answer.
   - Listen, but do not give yourself the answer. Do not tell yourself the answer; listen for it.
   - Continue asking on each in-breath for some time. If no answer comes, try again another time.

6. ❑ **Attending to your breath coming in and out, let your attention settle into your center.**

   - Breathing in completely, notice and follow the sensations of your breath coming in.
   - Let your attention settle into your center, at the bottom of your breath, at your solar plexus—*or*
   - Let your attention settle in the center of your forehead, your "third eye," at the top of your breath.
   - Keeping your attention at your center, exhale, breathing normally, maintaining attention.
   - Settle into Wise Mind.

7. ❑ **Expanding awareness.** Breathing in, focus your awareness on your center.

   - Breathing out, stay aware of your center, but expand awareness to the space you are in now.
   - Continue on in the moment.

8. ❑ **Dropping into the pauses between inhaling and exhaling.**

   - Breathing in, notice the pause after inhaling (top of breath).
   - Breathing out, notice the pause after exhaling (bottom of breath).
   - At each pause, let yourself "fall into" the center space within the pause.

9. ❑ **Other Wise Mind practice ideas:** _____

_____

_____

_____

_____

Taking Hold of Your Mind: "What" Skills

OBSERVE

❑ **Notice your body sensations** (coming through your eyes, ears, nose, skin, and tongue).

❑ **Pay attention** on purpose, to the present moment.

❑ **Control your attention,** but not what you see. Push away nothing. Cling to nothing.

❑ **Practice wordless watching:** Watch thoughts come into your mind and let them slip right by like clouds in the sky. Notice each feeling, rising and falling, like waves in the ocean.

❑ **Observe both inside and outside yourself.**

DESCRIBE

❑ **Put words on the experience.** When a feeling or thought arises, or you do something, acknowledge it. For example, say in your mind, "Sadness has just enveloped me," or "Stomach muscles tightening," or "A thought 'I can't do this' has come into my mind."

❑ **Label what you observe.** Put a name on your feelings. Label a thought as just a thought, a feeling as just a feeling, an action as just an action.

❑ **Unglue your interpretations and opinions** from the facts. Describe the "who, what, when, and where" that you observe. Just the facts.

❑ Remember, **If you can't observe it through your senses, you can't describe it.**

PARTICIPATE

❑ **Throw yourself completely into activities of the current moment.** Do not separate yourself from what is going on in the moment (dancing, cleaning, talking to a friend, feeling happy or feeling sad).

❑ **Become one with whatever you are doing,** completely forgetting yourself. Throw your attention to the moment.

❑ **Act intuitively from Wise Mind.** Do just what is needed in each situation—a skillful dancer on the dance floor, one with the music and your partner, neither willful nor sitting on your hands.

❑ **Go with the flow.** Respond with spontaneity.

Ideas for Practicing Observing

BY COMING BACK TO YOUR SENSES

Remember: Observing is bringing your mind back to the sensations of your body and mind.

Observe with your eyes:

1. ❑ Lie on the ground and watch the clouds in the sky.
2. ❑ Walking slowly, stopping somewhere with a view, notice flowers, trees, and nature itself.
3. ❑ Sit outside. Watch who and what go by in front of you, without following them with your head or your eyes.
4. ❑ Notice the facial expression and movements of another person. Refrain from labeling the person's emotions, thoughts, or interests.
5. ❑ Notice just the eyes, lips, or hands of another person (or just one feature of an animal).
6. ❑ Pick up a leaf, a flower, or a pebble. Look at it closely, trying to see each detail.
7. ❑ Find something beautiful to look at, and spend a few minutes contemplating it.
8. Other: _____

Observe sounds:

9. ❑ Stop for a moment and just listen. Listen to the texture and shape of the sounds around you. Listen to the silences between the sounds.
10. ❑ If someone is talking, listen to the pitch of the voice, to the smoothness or roughness of the sounds, to the clarity or the mumbling of the speech, to the pauses between the words.
11. ❑ Listen to music, observing each note as it comes and the spaces between the notes. Try breathing the sounds into your body and letting them flow out again on your out breath.
12. Other: _____

Observe smells around you:

13. ❑ Breathing in, notice any smells around you. Bring something close to your nose, and notice the smells. Take it away, and then notice the smells again. Do they linger?
14. ❑ When eating, notice the aroma of the food; when cooking, notice the aroma of the spices or other ingredients; when bathing, smell the soap or shampoo; when walking outside, notice the aroma of the air; when near flowers, bend down and "smell the roses."
15. Other: _____

Observe taste and the act of eating:

16. ❑ Putting something in your mouth, pay attention to the taste. Keep it in your mouth, and notice all the taste sensations.
17. ❑ Lick a lollipop or something else. Notice just the sensation of taste.
18. ❑ Eat a meal, or even a part of a meal, paying attention to the taste of each mouthful.
19. Other: _____

Observe urges to do something:

When you are feeling an urge to do something impulsive,

20. ❑ "Urge-surf" by imagining that your urges are a surfboard and you are standing on the board, riding the waves.
21. ❑ Notice any urge to avoid someone or something.
22. ❑ Scan your entire body, and notice the sensations. Where in the body is the urge?
23. ❑ When you are chewing your food, notice when you have the urge to swallow.
24. Other: _____

(*continued on next page*)

Observe sensations of touch on your skin:

25. ❑ Stroke your upper lip with your fingernail.
    - Stop stroking, and notice how long it takes before you can't sense your upper lip at all.
26. ❑ When walking, notice the sensations of walking—your feet hitting the ground and rising up and down. Sometimes walk very slowly and notice. Sometimes walk very fast and notice.
27. ❑ When sitting, notice your thighs on the chair. Notice the curve of your knees and your back.
28. ❑ Pay attention to anything touching you.
    - Try to feel your feet in your shoes, your body touching your clothes.
    - Feel your arms touching a chair.
    - Notice the sensations of your hands.
29. ❑ Touch something—the wall, a fabric, a table top, a pet, a piece of fruit, a person.
    - Notice the texture of what you feel, notice the sensations on your skin.
    - Try it again with another part of your body.
    - Notice the sensations again.
30. ❑ Focus your attention on the sensations in your chest, your stomach, or your shoulders.
31. ❑ Focus your attention on the place in your body where you feel tight or tense.
32. ❑ Focus your attention on the space between your eyes.
33. Other: _____

Observe your breath: *Breathe evenly and gently, focusing your attention on:*

34. ❑ The movement of your stomach.
    - As you begin to breathe in, allow your belly to rise in order to bring air into the lower half of your lungs.
    - As the upper halves of your lungs begin to fill with air, your chest begins to rise.
    - As you breathe out, notice your belly, then notice your chest. Don't tire yourself.
35. ❑ The pauses in your breathing.
    - As you breathe in, notice the brief pause when your lungs have filled with air.
    - As you breathe out, notice the brief pause when you have expelled all the air.
36. ❑ The sensations in your nose as you breathe in and as you breathe out.
    - As you breathe, close your mouth and breathe in through your nose, noticing the sensations traveling up and down your nostrils.
37. ❑ Your breath while walking slowly. Breathe normally.
    - Determine the length of your breath—the exhalation and the inhalation—by the number of your footsteps. Continue for a few minutes.
    - Begin to lengthen your exhalation by one step. Do not force a longer inhalation. Let it be natural.
    - Watch your inhalation carefully to see whether there is a desire to lengthen it. Now lengthen the exhalation by one more footstep.
    - Watch to see whether the inhalation also lengthens by one step or not.
    - Only lengthen the inhalation when you feel that it will be comfortable.
    - After 20 breaths, return your breath to normal.
38. ❑ Your breath while listening to a piece of music.
    - Breathe long, light, and even breaths.
    - Follow your breath; be master of it, while remaining aware of the movement and sentiments of the music.
    - Do not get lost in the music, but continue to be master of your breath and yourself.
39. ❑ Your breath while listening to a friend's words and your own replies. Continue as with music.
40. Other: _____

(*continued on next page*)

Observe thoughts coming in and out of your mind:

41. ❑ Notice thoughts as they come into your mind.
    - Ask, "Where do thoughts come from?"
    - Then watch them to see if you can see where they come into your mind.
42. ❑ As you notice thoughts in your mind, notice the pauses between each thought.
43. ❑ Imagine that your mind is the sky and that thoughts are clouds.
    - Notice each thought-cloud as it drifts by, letting it drift in and out of your mind.
    - Imagine thoughts as leaves on water flowing down a stream, as boats drifting by on the lake, or as train cars rolling by you.
44. ❑ When worries go round and round in your mind, move your attention to the sensations in your body (those most intense right now). Then, keeping your attention on your body sensations, notice how long it takes for the worries to ooze away.
45. ❑ Step back from your mind, as if you are on top of a mountain and your mind is just a boulder down below.
    - Gaze at your mind, watching what thoughts come up when you are watching it.
    - Come back into your mind before you stop.
46. ❑ Watch for the first two thoughts that come into your mind.
47. Other: _____

Imagine that your mind is a:

48. ❑ Conveyor belt, and that thoughts and feelings are coming down the belt.
    - Put each thought or feeling in a box, and then put it on the conveyor belt and let it go by.
49. ❑ Conveyor belt, and that you are sorting thoughts and feelings as they come down the belt.
    - Label the types of thoughts or feelings coming by (e.g., worry thoughts, thoughts about my past, thoughts about my mother, planning-what-to-do thoughts, angry feeling, sad feelings).
    - Put them in boxes nearby for another time.
50. ❑ River, and that thoughts and feelings are boats going down the river.
    - Imagine sitting on the grass, watching the boats go by.
    - Describe or label each boat as it goes by.
    - Try not to jump on the boat.
51. ❑ Railroad track, and that thoughts and feelings are train cars going by.
    - Describe or label each as it goes by. Try not to jump on the train.
52. Other: _____

Observe by expanding awareness:

53. ❑ Breathing in, notice your breath. Then, keeping your breath in your awareness, on the next breath notice your hands. Then, keeping both in your awareness, on the next breath expand your awareness to sounds.
    - Continue holding all three in awareness at the same time.
    - Practice this awareness of threes at other times, selecting other things to be aware of.
54. ❑ Keeping your focus on what you are currently doing, gently expand your awareness to include the space around you.
55. ❑ Go hug a tree, and feel the sensations of the embrace.
    - Attend to the embrace of the sheets and blankets or comforters around you as you lie in bed.
    - Do this when you feel lonely and want to be loved or to love.
56. Other: _____

(*continued on next page*)

Open your mind to your senses:

57. ❑ Practice walking with your senses as wide open as you can make them.
    - Notice what you hear, see, and feel.
    - Notice what you feel when shifting your weight between each step.
    - Notice your body experience as you turn.

58. ❑ For one mouthful in a meal, pause with a spoonful or forkful of food.
    - Look at what you are going to eat, smell it, and listen to it. Then, when you are ready, put it in your mouth.
    - Note the taste, texture, temperature, and even the sound your teeth make in chewing your mouthful slowly.
    - Note the changes in its taste, texture, temperature, and sound as you chew it to completion.

59. ❑ Focus your mind on paying attention to each sensation that comes into your mind.
    - Attend to sensations of sight, smell, touch, hearing, and taste, or to the thoughts generated by your brain.
    - Notice sensations as they arise, and notice them as they fall away.
    - Let your mind focus on each sensation as it arises.
    - Notice each sensation with curiosity, allowing it to be. Examine the uniqueness of each sensation.

60. ❑ Be here. Be in the present now.
    - Take a moment to notice every sense you are aware of.
    - To yourself, make a statement, about each sense: "I feel the chair; the chair feels me." "I hear the heater; the heater hears me." "I see the wall; the wall sees me." "I hear a stomach growl; it hears me."

61. ❑ When a feeling arises within you, notice it—saying, for example, "A feeling of sadness is arising within me."

62. ❑ When a thought arises within you, notice it—saying, for example, "The thought 'It is hot in here' is arising within me."

63. ❑ Take just a moment of your time, and practice "nothing-to-do" mind.
    - Let yourself become completely aware of your present experience, noticing sensations and the space around you.

64. ❑ Find a small object, one you can hold in your hand. Place it in front of you on a table or in your lap. Observe it closely—first not moving it, and then picking it up and turning it over and around, gazing at it from different angles and in different lights. Just notice shapes, colors, sizes, and other characteristics that are visible.
    - Then change your focus to your fingers and hands touching the object. Notice the sensations of touching the object; notice the texture, temperature, and feel of the object.
    - Put the object down. Close your eyes, and inhale and exhale deeply and slowly.
    - Then, with beginner's mind, open your eyes. With new vision, once again notice the object. With beginner's mind, open to feeling new textures and sensations, explore the object with your fingers and hands.
    - Put down the object, and once again focus your mind on inhaling and exhaling once.

65. Other: _____

Ideas for Practicing Describing

Practice describing what you see outside of yourself:

1. ❑ Lie on the ground and watch the clouds in the sky. Find and describe cloud patterns that you see.

2. ❑ Sit on a bench on a busy street or at a park. Describe one thing about each person who walks by you.

3. ❑ Find things in nature—a leaf, a drop of water, a pet or other animal. Describe each thing in as much detail as you can.

4. ❑ Describe as accurately as you can what a person has just said to you. Check to see if you are correct.

5. ❑ Describe a person's face when the person seems angry, afraid, or sad. Notice and describe the shape, movement, and placement of the forehead, eyebrows, and eyes; the lips and mouth; the cheeks; and so on.

6. ❑ Describe what a person has done or is doing now. Be very specific. Avoid describing intentions or outcomes of the behavior that you do not directly observe. Avoid judgmental language.

7. Other: _____

Practice describing thoughts and feelings:

8. ❑ Describe your feelings as they arise within you: "A feeling of anger is arising within me."

9. ❑ Describe your thoughts when you feel a strong emotion: "I feel X, and my thoughts are Y."

10. ❑ Describe your feelings after someone else does or says something: "When you do X, I feel Y."

11. ❑ Describe thoughts, feelings, and what you observed others do: "When you do X, I feel Y, and my thoughts are Z." "When X occurs, I feel Y, and my thoughts are Z."

12. ❑ Describe as many of your thoughts as you can while feeling a strong emotion.

13. Other: _____

Practice describing your breathing:

14. ❑ Each time you inhale and exhale, as you inhale, be aware that "I am inhaling, 1." When you exhale, be aware that "I am exhaling, 1." Remember to breathe from the stomach. When beginning the second inhalation, be aware that "I am inhaling, 2." And, slowly exhaling, be aware that "I am exhaling, 2." Continue on up through 10. After you have reached 10, return to 1. Whenever you lose count, return to 1.

15. ❑ Begin to inhale gently and normally (from the stomach), describing in your mind that "I am inhaling normally." Exhale in awareness, "I am exhaling normally." Continue for three breaths. On the fourth breath, extend the inhalation, describing in your mind that "I am breathing in a long inhalation." Exhale in awareness, "I am breathing out a long exhalation." Continue for three breaths.

16. ❑ Follow the entrance and exit of air. Say to yourself, "I am inhaling and following the inhalation from its beginning to its end. I am exhaling and following the exhalation from its beginning to its end."

17. Other: _____

Ideas for Practicing Participating

Participate with awareness of connection to the universe:

1. ❑ Focus your attention on where your body touches an object (floor or ground, air molecules, a chair or armrest, your bed sheets and covers, your clothes, etc.). Try to see all the ways you are connected to and accepted by that object. Consider the function of that object with relation to you. That is, consider what the object does for you. Consider its kindness in doing that. Experience the sensation of touching the object, and focus your entire attention on that kindness until a sense of being connected or loved or cared for arises in your heart.

   Examples: Focus your attention on your feet touching the ground. Consider the kindness of the ground holding you up, providing a path for you to get to other things, not letting you fall away from everything else. Focus your attention on your body touching the chair you sit in. Consider how the chair accepts you totally, holds you up, supports your back, and keeps you from falling down on the floor. Focus your attention on the sheets and covers on your bed. Consider the touch of the sheets and covers holding you, surrounding and keeping you warm and comfortable. Consider the walls in the room. They keep out the wind and the cold and the rain. Think of how the walls are connected to you via the floor and the air in the room. Experience your connection to the walls that provide you with a secure place to do things. Go hug a tree. Think of how you and the tree are connected. Life is in you and in the tree and both of you are warmed by the sun, held by the air and supported by the earth. Try and experience the tree loving you by providing something to lean on, or by shading you.

2. ❑ Dance to music.

3. ❑ Sing along with music you are listening to.

4. ❑ Sing in the shower.

5. ❑ Sing and dance while watching TV.

6. ❑ Jump out of bed and dance, or sing before getting dressed.

7. ❑ Go to a church that sings, and join in the singing.

8. ❑ Play karaoke with friends or at a karaoke club or bar.

9. ❑ Throw yourself into what another person is saying.

10. ❑ Go running, focusing only on running.

11. ❑ Play a sport and throw yourself into playing.

12. ❑ Become the count of the breath, becoming only "one" when you count 1, becoming only "two" when you count 2, and so on.

13. ❑ Become a word as you slowly say the word over and over and over.

14. ❑ Take a class in improvisational acting.

15. ❑ Take a dance class.

16. Other: _____

Taking Hold of Your Mind: "How" Skills

NONJUDGMENTALLY

☐ **See, but don't evaluate as good or bad.** Just the facts.

☐ **Accept each moment like a blanket spread out on the lawn,** accepting both the rain and the sun and each leaf that falls upon it.

☐ **Acknowledge** the difference between the helpful and the harmful, the safe and the dangerous, **but don't judge them.**

☐ **Acknowledge** your values, your wishes, your emotional reactions, **but don't judge them.**

☐ When you find yourself judging, **don't judge your judging.**

ONE-MINDFULLY

☐ **Rivet yourself to now.** Be completely present to this one moment.

☐ **Do one thing at a time.** Notice the desire to be half-present, to be somewhere else, to go somewhere else in your mind, to do something else, to multitask—and then come back to one thing at a time.

- When you are eating, eat.
- When you are walking, walk.
- When you are worrying, worry.
- When you are planning, plan.
- When you are remembering, remember.

☐ **Let go of distractions.** If other actions, or other thoughts, or strong feelings distract you, go back to what you are doing—again, and again, and again.

☐ **Concentrate your mind.** If you find you are doing two things at once, stop—go back to one thing at a time (the opposite of multitasking!).

EFFECTIVELY

☐ **Be mindful of your goals in the situation,** and do what is necessary to achieve them.

☐ **Focus on what works.** (Don't let emotion mind get in the way of being effective.)

☐ **Play by the rules.**

☐ **Act as skillfully as you can.** Do what is needed for the situation you are in—not the situation you wish you were in; not the one that is fair; not the one that is more comfortable.

☐ **Let go of willfulness and sitting on your hands.**

Ideas for Practicing Nonjudgmentalness

Leaving out comparisons, judgments, and assumptions:

1. ❑ Practice observing judgmental thoughts and statements, saying in your mind, **"A judgmental thought arose in my mind."**

2. ❑ **Count judgmental thoughts and statements** (by moving objects or pieces of paper from one pocket to another, by clicking a sports counter, or by marking a piece of paper).

3. ❑ Replace judgmental thoughts and statements with nonjudgmental thoughts and statements.

   Tips for replacing judgment by stating the facts:

   1. **Describe the facts** of the event or situation—*only* what is observed with your senses.

   2. **Describe the consequences** of the event. Keep to the facts.

   3. **Describe your own feelings** in response to the facts (remember, emotions are not judgments).

4. ❑ **Observe your judgmental facial expressions, postures, and voice tones** (including voice tones in your head).

5. ❑ **Change judgmental expressions, postures, and voice tones.**

6. ❑ Tell someone what you did today nonjudgmentally, or about an event that occurred. Stay very concrete; only relate what you observed directly.

7. ❑ **Write out a nonjudgmental description** of an event that prompted an emotion.

8. ❑ Write out a nonjudgmental blow-by-blow account of a particularly important episode in your day. Describe both what happened in your environment and what your thoughts, feelings, and actions were. Leave out any analysis of why something happened, or why you thought, felt, or acted as you did. Stick to the facts that you observed.

9. ❑ Imagine a person you are angry with. Bring to mind what the person has done that has caused so much anger. Try to become that person, seeing life from that person's point of view. Imagine that person's feelings, thoughts, fears, hopes, and wishes. Imagine that person's history and what has happened in his or her history. Imagine understanding that person.

10. ❑ When judgmental, **practice half-smiling and/or willing hands.** (See Distress Tolerance Handout 14: Half-Smiling and Willing Hands.)

11. Other: _____

Ideas for Practicing One-Mindfulness

1. ☐ **Awareness while making tea or coffee.** Prepare a pot of tea or coffee to serve a guest or to drink by yourself. Do each movement slowly, in awareness. Do not let one detail of your movements go by without being aware of it. Know that your hand lifts the pot by its handle. Know that you are pouring the fragrant, warm tea or coffee into the cup. Follow each step in awareness. Breathe gently and more deeply than usual. Take hold of your breath if your mind strays.

2. ☐ **Awareness while washing the dishes.** Wash the dishes consciously, as though each bowl is an object of contemplation. Consider each bowl sacred. Follow your breath to prevent your mind from straying. Do not try to hurry to get the job over with. Consider washing the dishes the most important thing in life.

3. ☐ **Awareness while hand-washing clothes.** Do not wash too many clothes at one time. Select only three or four articles of clothing. Find the most comfortable position to sit or stand, so as to prevent a backache. Scrub the clothes consciously. Hold your attention on every movement of your hands and arms. Pay attention to the soap and water. When you have finished scrubbing and rinsing, your mind and body will feel as clean and fresh as your clothes. Remember to maintain a half-smile and take hold of your breath whenever your mind wanders.

4. ☐ **Awareness while cleaning house.** Divide your work into stages: straightening things and putting away books, scrubbing the toilet, scrubbing the bathroom, sweeping the floors, and dusting. Allow a good length of time for each task. Move slowly, three times more slowly than usual. Focus your attention fully on each task. For example, while placing a book on the shelf, look at the book; be aware of what book it is; know that you are in the process of placing it on the shelf; and know that you intend to put it in that specific place. Know that your hand reaches for the book and picks it up. Avoid any abrupt or harsh movement. Maintain awareness of the breath, especially when your thoughts wander.

5. ☐ **Awareness while taking a slow-motion bath.** Allow yourself 30–45 minutes to take a bath. Don't hurry for even a second. From the moment you prepare the bath water to the moment you put on clean clothes, let every motion be light and slow. Be attentive of every movement. Place your attention on every part of your body, without discrimination or fear. Be aware of each stream of water on your body. By the time you've finished, your mind will feel as peaceful and light as your body. Follow your breath. Think of yourself as being in a clean and fragrant lotus pond in the summer.

6. ☐ **Awareness with meditation.** Sit comfortably on the floor with your back straight, on the floor or in a chair with both feet touching the floor. Close your eyes all the way, or open them slightly and gaze at something near. With each breath, say to yourself, quietly and gently, the word "One." As you inhale, say the word "One." As you exhale, say the word "One," calmly and slowly. Try to collect your whole mind and put it into this one word. When your mind strays, return gently to saying "One." If you start wanting to move, try not to move. Just gently observe wanting to move. Continue practicing a little past wanting to stop. Just gently observe wanting to stop.

7. Other: _____

Ideas for Practicing Effectiveness

1. ❑ Observe when you begin to get angry or hostile with someone. Ask yourself, "Is this effective?"

2. ❑ Observe yourself when you start wanting to be "right" instead of effective. Give up being "right" and switch to trying to be effective.

3. ❑ Notice willfulness in yourself. Ask yourself, "Is this effective?"

4. ❑ Drop willfulness, and practice acting effectively instead. Notice the difference.

5. ❑ When feeling angry or hostile or like you're about to do something ineffective, practice willing hands.

6. Other: _____

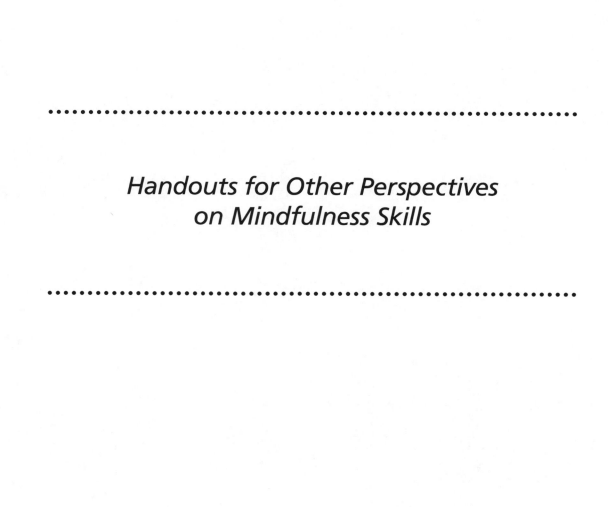

*Handouts for Other Perspectives
on Mindfulness Skills*

Overview:
Other Perspectives on Mindfulness

MINDFULNESS PRACTICE:

A Spiritual Perspective

SKILLFUL MEANS:

Taking hold of your everyday life by balancing Doing Mind and Being Mind

---

WISE MIND:

Walking the Middle Path

Goals of Mindfulness Practice:
A Spiritual Perspective

TO EXPERIENCE:

❑ Ultimate reality *as it is* which leads to a sense of inner spaciousness and awareness of intimate wholeness with the entire universe, the transcendence of boundaries, and the ground of our being.

❑ Other: _____

TO GROW IN WISDOM:

❑ Of the heart and of action.

❑ Other: _____

TO EXPERIENCE FREEDOM:

❑ By letting go of attachments to the demands of your own desires, cravings, and intense emotions, and radically accepting reality as it is.

❑ Other: _____

TO INCREASE LOVE AND COMPASSION:

❑ Toward yourself.

❑ Toward others.

❑ Other: _____

❑ **Other:** _____

Wise Mind from a Spiritual Perspective

Wise Mind as . . . **Contemplative practice** Mindfulness Meditation Contemplative prayer Contemplative action Centering prayer	Thoughts, attitudes, and actions designed to help us express or experience connection to: • The sacred, the divine within, the transcendent. • God, the Great Spirit, the Absolute, Elohim, the nameless one, Brahma, Allah, Parvardigar. • Ultimate reality, the totality, the source, our essential nature, our true self, the core of our being, the ground of being. • No self, emptiness.
Wise Mind experience from a spiritual perspective	Experience where a deeper layer of reality rises to consciousness. A reality that has always been there but has been misperceived. An experience of expansion of consciousness; the experience of unity and oneness within the sacred.
Wise Mind **from the perspective of mysticism** (seven characteristics of mystical experiences)	1. **Direct experience:** Experience without words of *ultimate reality.* 2. **Experience of unity:** Awareness of oneness and of no distance between oneself, reality, and all other beings. 3. **Without words:** Experience of reality that cannot be grasped and can only be described with metaphors and stories. 4. **Certain:** During the experience, certainty of the experience is total, undeniable, clear. 5. **Practical:** Experience that is concretely beneficial to one's life and well-being. 6. **Integrative:** Experience that establishes harmony of love, compassion, mercy, kindness; quieting of extreme emotions. 7. **Sapiential:** Experience that leads to wisdom, enhances capacity for intuitive knowledge.

Practicing Loving Kindness to Increase Love and Compassion

WHAT IS LOVING KINDNESS?

Loving kindness is a mindfulness practice designed to increase love and compassion first for ourselves and then for our loved ones, for friends, for those we are angry with, for difficult people, for enemies, and then for all beings.

Loving kindness can protect us from developing and holding on to judgmentalness, ill will, and hostile feelings toward ourselves and others.

PRACTICING LOVING KINDNESS

Practicing loving kindness is like saying a prayer for yourself or someone else. As when you are asking or praying for something for yourself or others, you actively send loving and kind wishes, and recite in your mind words and phrases that express good will toward yourself and others.

LOVING KINDNESS INSTRUCTIONS

1. Choose a person to send loving kindness toward. Do *not* select a person you do not want to relate to with kindness and compassion. Start with yourself, or, if this is too difficult, with a person you already love.

2. Sitting, standing, or lying down, begin by breathing slowly and deeply. Opening the palms of your hands, gently bring the person to mind.

3. Radiate loving kindness by reciting a set of warm wishes, such as "May I be happy," "May I be at peace," "May I be healthy," "May I be safe," or another set of positive wishes of your own. Repeat the script slowly, and focus on the meaning of each word as you say it in your mind. (If you have distracting thoughts, just notice them as they come and go and gently bring your mind back to your script.) Continue until you feel yourself immersed in loving kindness.

4. Gradually work yourself up through loved ones, friends, those you are angry with, difficult people, enemies, and finally all beings. For example, use a script such as "May John be happy," "May John be at peace," and so on (or "John, may you be happy," "May you be at peace," and so on), as you concentrate on radiating loving kindness to John.

5. Practice each day, starting with yourself and then moving to others.

Skillful Means:
Balancing Doing Mind and Being Mind

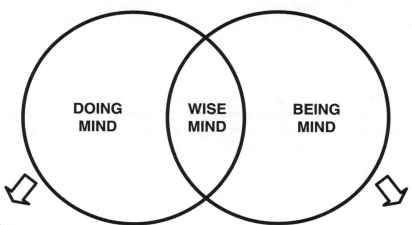

Doing Mind Is:

- **Discriminating Mind**

- **Ambitious Mind**

- **Goal-Oriented**

When in *doing mind,* you view your thoughts as facts about the world. You are focused on problem solving and achieving goals.

Wise Mind Is:

- A balance of doing and being

- The middle path

When in Wise Mind, you:

Use skillful means.

Let go of having to achieve goals—and throw your entire self into working toward these same goals.

Enhance awareness while engaging in activities.

Being Mind Is:

- **Curious Mind**

- **Nothing-to-Do Mind**

- **Present-Oriented**

When in *being mind,* you view your thoughts as sensations of the mind. You are focused on the uniqueness of each moment, letting go of focusing on goals.

Note. The terms "doing mind," "being mind," and "nothing-to-do mind" were first used by Jon Kabat-Zinn in *Full Catastrophe Living* (1990, 2013).

Ideas for Practicing Balancing
Doing Mind and Being Mind

The mindfulness skills require a lot of practice. The practice ideas below are to help you act skillfully in everyday life, bringing together doing activities of everyday life with being mind.

1. ❑ **Wise Mind reading.** To increase your desire for mindfulness, find readings or quotations that have the effect of making you actually want to practice mindfulness in your everyday life. Put these quotations at strategic spots in your life (e.g., near the coffee maker), and then while you are waiting for other things, read the inspirational messages.

2. ❑ **Wise Mind reminders.** Set an alarm at home, at work, or (if possible) on your cell phone or watch to go off randomly or at set times. Use the alarm as a reminder to be mindful of your current activities. (See *www.mindfulnessdc.org/bell/index.html* or a similar Internet site for a free mindfulness clock to download onto your computer.) Set up automatic text messages or Twitter messages to remind yourself. Write out mindfulness quotations that you like, and tape them in strategic places where you will see them as reminders to practice mindfulness.

3. ❑ **Wise Mind in the routine of daily life.** Choose one routine activity in your daily life (such as brushing your teeth, getting dressed, making coffee or tea, working on a task). Make a deliberate effort to bring moment-to-moment awareness to that activity.

4. ❑ **"Just this one moment" Wise Mind.** When you begin to feel overwhelmed or frazzled, say, "Just this one moment, just this one task," to remind yourself that your only requirement at the moment is to do one thing in the moment—wash one dish, take one step, move one set of muscles. In this moment, let the next moment go until you get there.

(*continued on next page*)

Note. Exercises 3 and 4 are from Segal, Z. V., Williams, J. M. G., & Teasdale, J. D. (2013). *Mindfulness-based cognitive therapy for depression: A new approach to preventing relapse* (2nd ed.). New York: Guilford Press. Copyright 2013 by The Guilford Press. Adapted by permission. All other exercises are adapted from Kabat-Zinn, J. (1990). *Full catastrophe living: Using the wisdom of your body and mind to face stress, pain, and illness.* New York: Delacorte Press. Copyright 1990 by Jon Kabat-Zinn. Adapted by permission of Random House.

5. ❑ **Wise Mind awareness of events.** Notice events in your everyday life (both pleasant and unpleasant), even if they are only very small (such as warm water on your hands when washing, the taste of something you eat, the feel of wind on your face, the fact that your car is running out of gas or that you are tired).

6. ❑ **Wise Mind awareness of what needs to be done.** When relaxing after a hard day's work or at a break during the day, stay aware of what needs to be done and focus on doing what is needed.

7. ❑ **Wise Mind willingness.** Practice willingness to do what is needed when you are asked, or when you see that something needs to be done. Do what is needed with a balance of being and doing, focusing the mind, immersing yourself in the task.

8. ❑ **Three-minute WISE MIND: Slowing down "doing mind" in your everyday life**

   • Bring yourself into the present moment by adopting a "wide-awake" posture, and then, in Wise Mind, ask, "What is my experience right now? What thoughts and images are going through my mind?" Notice them as mental events, as neural firing in your brain. Next ask, "What are my feelings and sensations in my body?" Notice these as they come into your awareness. Then say, "OK, this is how it is right now."

   • Settle into Wise Mind and focus your entire attention on your breath as it goes in and as it goes out, one breath after another. Gather yourself all together, and focus on the movements of your chest and abdomen, the rise and fall of your breath, moment by moment, breath by breath as best you can. Let your breath become an anchor to bring you into the present moment.

   • Once you have gathered yourself to some extent, allow your awareness to expand. As well as being aware of the breath, include also a sense of the body as a whole, your posture, your facial expression, your hands. Follow the breath as if your whole body is breathing. When you are ready, step back into your activities, acting from Wise Mind of your whole body in the present moment.

9. ❑ **Other Wise Mind practice ideas:** _____

Walking the Middle Path:
Finding the Synthesis between Opposites

**Reasonable
mind** ←——————————△——————————→ **Emotion
mind**

Both regulate actions and make decisions based on reason,
And
take into account values and experience even strong emotions as they come and go.

**Doing
mind** ←——————————△——————————→ **Nothing-to-do
mind**

Both do what is needed in the moment (including reviewing the past or planning for the future),
And
experience fully the uniqueness of each moment in the moment.

**Intense desire
for change
of the moment** ←——————————△——————————→ **Radical
acceptance
of the moment**

Both allow yourself to have an intense desire to have something else than what is now,
And
be willing to radically accept what you have in your life in the present moment.

Self-denial ←——————————△——————————→ **Self-indulgence**

Both practice moderation,
And
satisfy the senses.

Other:

_____   _____
←——————————△——————————→
_____   _____

Mindfulness Worksheets

*Worksheets for Core
Mindfulness Skills*

Pros and Cons of Practicing Mindfulness

Due Date: _____   Name: _____ Week Starting: _____

Make a list of the pros and cons of practicing mindfulness skills.
Make another list of the pros and cons of *not* practicing mindfulness skills.
Check the facts to be sure that you are correct in your assessment of advantages and disadvantages.

Rate Willingness to Practice (0 = None; 100 = Very High)   **Before:** _____   **After:** _____

Fill this worksheet out when you are:
- Trying to decide whether to work on becoming more mindful of the moments in your life.
- Feeling willful; saying no to letting go of emotion mind or extreme reasonable mind.
- Resisting observing the present moment, rather than escaping it or trying to control it.
- Resisting giving up your interpretations of others or yourself, rather than just describing.
- Resisting throwing yourself into the flow of the moment; wanting to stand on the outside.
- Feeling threatened whenever you think of letting go of judgments.
- Not in the mood for being effective instead of proving you are right.

When you are filling out this worksheet, think about these questions:
- Is a mindless life in your best interest (i.e., effective), or not in your best interest (i.e., ineffective)?
- Will refusing to go into Wise Mind solve a problem, or make a new problem for you?
- Is observing the moment without reacting to it immediately likely to increase your freedom, or decrease it?
- Is being attached to your thoughts instead of the facts you can describe useful, or not?
- Is staying judgmental helping you change the things you want to change, or getting in the way?
- Is it more important to be effective, or to be right?

	Stay Mindless, Judgmental, Ineffective	**Practice Mindfulness**
PROS	_____ _____ _____ _____ _____	_____ _____ _____ _____ _____
CONS	_____ _____ _____ _____ _____	_____ _____ _____ _____ _____

What did you decide to do? _____
Is this the best decision (in Wise Mind)? _____
List any and all wise things you did this week. _____

Mindfulness Core Skills Practice

Due Date: _____ Name: _____ Week Starting: _____

Describe the situations that prompted you to practice mindfulness.

SITUATION 1

Situation (who, what, when, where):

❑ Wise Mind
❑ Observe
❑ Describe
❑ Participate
❑ Nonjudgmentally
❑ One-mindfully
❑ Effectively

At left, check the skills you used, and describe your use of them here.

Describe experience of using the skill:

Check if practicing this mindfulness skill has influenced any of the following, *even a little bit:*

__Reduced suffering   __Increased happiness   __Increased ability to focus
__Decreased reactivity   __Increased wisdom   __Increased experiencing the
__Increased connection   __Increased sense of personal validity   present

SITUATION 2

Situation (who, what, when, where):

❑ Wise Mind
❑ Observe
❑ Describe
❑ Participate
❑ Nonjudgmentally
❑ One-mindfully
❑ Effectively

At left, check the skills you used, and describe your use of them here.

Describe experience of using the skill:

Check if practicing this mindfulness skill has influenced any of the following, *even a little bit:*

__Reduced suffering   __Increased happiness   __Increased ability to focus
__Decreased reactivity   __Increased wisdom   __Increased experiencing the
__Increased connection   __Increased sense of personal validity   present

List any and all wise things you did this week. _____

Mindfulness Core Skills Practice

Due Date: _____ Name: _____ Week Starting: _____

For each mindfulness skill, write down what you did during the week, and then rate the quality of mindfulness you experienced during your practice.

I could not focus my mind for even 1 second; I was completely mindless and quit.		*I was able to focus my mind somewhat and stay in the present moment.*		*I became centered in Wise Mind and was free to let go and do what was needed.*
1	**2**	**3**	**4**	**5**

Day **Wise Mind**

_____/_____ Mindfulness: _____

_____/_____ Mindfulness: _____

_____/_____ Mindfulness: _____

Day: **Observe**

_____/_____ Mindfulness: _____

_____/_____ Mindfulness: _____

_____/_____ Mindfulness: _____

Day: **Describe**

_____/_____ Mindfulness: _____

_____/_____ Mindfulness: _____

_____/_____ Mindfulness: _____

Day: **Participate**

_____/_____ Mindfulness: _____

_____/_____ Mindfulness: _____

_____/_____ Mindfulness: _____

Day: **Nonjudgmentally**

_____/_____ Mindfulness: _____

_____/_____ Mindfulness: _____

_____/_____ Mindfulness: _____

Day: **One-mindfully**

_____/_____ Mindfulness: _____

_____/_____ Mindfulness: _____

_____/_____ Mindfulness: _____

Day: **Effectively**

_____/_____ Mindfulness: _____

_____/_____ Mindfulness: _____

_____/_____ Mindfulness: _____

List any and all wise things you did this week. _____

(Mindfulness Handouts 2–5c)

Mindfulness Core Skills Practice

Due Date: _____ Name: _____ Week Starting: _____

Practice each mindfulness skill twice, and describe your experience as follows:

When did you practice this skill, and what did you do to practice?	What was going on that prompted practicing mindfulness (if anything)?	How much time passed when you were doing this skill?	Rate before/after skill use		Conclusions or questions about this skills practice
			Degree of focusing my mind (0–100)	Degree of being centered in Wise Mind (0–100)	
Wise Mind:			/	/	
Observe:			/	/	
Describe:			/	/	
Participate:			/	/	
Nonjudgmentally:			/	/	
One-mindfully:			/	/	
Effectively:			/	/	

List any and all wise things you did this week: _____

Note. Adapted from an unpublished worksheet by Seth Axelrod, with his permission.

Mindfulness Core Skills Calendar

Due Date: _____ Name: _____ Week Starting: _____

Check off skills to practice this week:

___ Wise Mind ___ Observing ___ Describing ___ Participating ___ Nonjudgmentally ___ One-mindfully ___ Effectively

While you are practicing skills, stay as aware and mindful as you can. Write it down later.

Name(s) of skill(s)	How did you practice the skill?	Describe your experience, including body sensations, emotions, and thoughts while practicing the skill	What is your experience now, after using the skill?
Example: *Participating*	*I went to a party and joined in conversations with other people.*	*I felt a tight knot in my stomach, shallow breathing, dry mouth, anxiety that other people would not like me; later I enjoyed the conversation, smiled, noticed other people around me, and ended up having a good time.*	*I feel amazed that I managed to do this and felt good about myself. I am thinking I may be able to do this again.*
Monday:			
Tuesday:			
Wednesday:			

(continued on next page)

Name(s) of skill(s)	How did you practice the skill?	Describe your experience, including body sensations, emotions, and thoughts while practicing the skill	What is your experience now, after using the skill?
Thursday:			
Friday:			
Saturday:			
Sunday:			

List any and all wise things you did this week: _____

Wise Mind Practice

Due Date: _____   Name: _____   Week Starting: _____

Wise Mind Practice Exercise: Check off an exercise each time you do one.

☐☐☐☐ **1.** Attended to my breath coming in and out, letting my attention settle into my center.

☐☐☐☐ **2.** Imagined being a flake of stone on the lake.

☐☐☐☐ **3.** Imagined walking down an inner spiral stairs.

☐☐☐☐ **4.** Dropped into the pauses between inhaling and exhaling.

☐☐☐☐ **5.** Breathed "wise" in, "mind" out.

☐☐☐☐ **6.** Asked Wise Mind a question (breathing in) and listened for the answer (breathing out).

☐☐☐☐ **7.** Asked myself, "Is this Wise Mind?"

☐☐☐☐ **8.** Other (describe): _____

☐☐☐☐ **9.** Other (describe): _____

Describe the situation and how you practiced Wise Mind:

_____

_____

How effective was the practice in helping you become centered in your Wise Mind?

Not effective: *I couldn't do the skill* *for even 1 minute. I got* *distracted or quit.*		*Somewhat effective:* *I was able to practice Wise Mind* *and became somewhat centered* *in my Wise Mind.*		*Very effective:* *I became centered in Wise* *Mind, and was free to do* *what needed to be done.*
1	**2**	**3**	**4**	**5**

Describe the situation and how you practiced Wise Mind:

_____

_____

How effective was the practice in helping you become centered in your Wise Mind?

Not effective: *I couldn't do the skill* *for even 1 minute. I got* *distracted or quit.*		*Somewhat effective:* *I was able to practice Wise Mind* *and became somewhat centered* *in my Wise Mind.*		*Very effective:* *I became centered in Wise* *Mind, and was free to do* *what needed to be done.*
1	**2**	**3**	**4**	**5**

List any and all wise things you did this week: _____

Mindfulness "What" Skills:
Observing, Describing, Participating

Due Date: _____   Name: _____ Week Starting: _____

Check off the mindfulness skills you practiced this week. Write out descriptions of two different times when you practiced a mindfulness skill. Use back of sheet for more examples.

____Observing   ____Describing   ____Participating

Describe the situation and how you practiced the skill:

_____

_____

_____

_____

Check if practicing this mindfulness skill has improved any of the following, *even a little bit*:

____Reduced suffering   ____Increased happiness   ____Increased ability to focus

____Decreased reactivity   ____Increased wisdom   ____Increased experiencing the present

____Increased connection   ____Increased sense of personal validity

Describe how the skill helped or did not help you become more mindful: _____

_____

Describe the situation and how you practiced the skill:

_____

_____

_____

_____

Check if practicing this mindfulness skill has improved any of the following, *even a little bit:*

____Reduced suffering   ____Increased happiness   ____Increased ability to focus

____Decreased reactivity   ____Increased wisdom   ____Increased experiencing the present

____Increased connection   ____Increased sense of personal validity

Describe how the skill helped or did not help you become more mindful: _____

_____

List any and all wise things you did this week: _____

Observing, Describing, Participating Checklist

Due Date: _____   Name: _____ Week Starting: _____

Check off mindfulness skills that you use when you use them. You can check each skill up to four times. If you practice a skill more than four times, extend your checks toward the edge of the page, or use the back of the page if needed.

Practice observing: Check off an exercise each time you do one.

☐☐☐☐ 1. What you see: ____Watch without following what you see.

☐☐☐☐ 2. Sounds: ____Sounds around you, ____pitch and sound of someone's voice, ____music.

☐☐☐☐ 3. Smells around you: ____Aroma of food, ____soap, ____air as you walk.

☐☐☐☐ 4. The taste of what you eat and the act of eating.

☐☐☐☐ 5. Urges to do something: ____Urge-surf, ____notice urge to avoid, ____notice where in body urge is.

☐☐☐☐ 6. Body sensations: ____Body scan, ____sensation of walking, ____body touching something.

☐☐☐☐ 7. Thoughts coming in and out of your mind: ____Imagine your mind as a river, ____as a conveyor belt.

☐☐☐☐ 8. Your breath: ____Movement of stomach, ____sensations of air in and out nose.

☐☐☐☐ 9. By expanding awareness: ____To your entire body, ____to space around you, ____to hugging a tree.

☐☐☐☐ 10. By opening the mind: ____To each sensation arising, not attaching, letting go of each.

☐☐☐☐ 11. Other (describe): _____

Practice describing: Check off an exercise each time you do one.

☐☐☐☐ 12. What you see outside of your body.

☐☐☐☐ 13. Thoughts, feelings, and body sensations inside yourself.

☐☐☐☐ 14. Your breathing.

☐☐☐☐ 15. Other (describe): _____

Practice participating: Check off an exercise each time you do one.

☐☐☐☐ 16. Dance to music.

☐☐☐☐ 17. Sing along with music you are listening to.

☐☐☐☐ 18. Sing in the shower.

☐☐☐☐ 19. Sing and dance while watching TV.

☐☐☐☐ 20. Jump out of bed and dance or sing before getting dressed.

☐☐☐☐ 21. Go to a church that sings and join in the singing.

☐☐☐☐ 22. Play karaoke with friends or at a karaoke club or bar.

☐☐☐☐ 23. Throw yourself into what another person is saying.

☐☐☐☐ 24. Go running, riding, skating, walking; become one with the activity.

☐☐☐☐ 25. Play a sport and throw yourself into playing.

☐☐☐☐ 26. Become the count of your breath, becoming only "one" when you count 1, becoming only "two" when you count 2, and so on.

☐☐☐☐ 27. Become a word as you slowly say the word over and over and over.

☐☐☐☐ 28. Throw caution to the wind, and throw yourself into a social or work activity.

☐☐☐☐ 29. Other (describe): _____

List any and all wise things you did this week: _____

Observing, Describing, Participating Calendar

Due Date: _____ Name: _____ Week Starting: _____

Check off at least two skills to practice this week: _____ Observing _____ Describing _____ Participating

While you are practicing skills, stay as aware and mindful as you can. Write it down later.

Name(s) of skill(s)	How did you practice the skill?	Describe your experience, including body sensations, emotions, and thoughts while practicing the skill	What is your experience now, after using the skill?
Example: *Observing*	*I took a walk in the park and observed the trees I encountered.*	*I felt calm, my shoulders relaxed. I felt curiosity toward the trees I was observing, a sense of detachment from my own worries; I thought the leaves of the trees were very green and refreshing.*	*I feel somewhat relaxed; I think I should go for walks more often. I am anxious that next time I might not be able to pay attention to the practice.*
Monday:			
Tuesday:			
Wednesday:			

(continued on next page)

Name(s) of skill(s)	How did you practice the skill?	Describe your experience, including body sensations, emotions, and thoughts while practicing the skill	What is your experience now, after using the skill?
Thursday:			
Friday:			
Saturday:			
Sunday:			

List any and all wise things you did this week: _____

Mindfulness "How" Skills:
Nonjudgmentalness, One-Mindfulness, Effectiveness

Due Date: _____ Name: _____ Week Starting: _____

Check off the mindfulness skills you practiced this week. Write out descriptions of two different times when you practiced a mindfulness skill. Use back of sheet for more examples.

____Nonjudgmentalness ____One-mindfulness ____Effectiveness

Describe the situation and how you practiced the skill:

_____

_____

_____

_____

Check if practicing this mindfulness skill has improved any of the following, *even a little bit*:

____Reduced suffering ____Increased happiness ____Increased ability to focus

____Decreased reactivity ____Increased wisdom ____Increased experiencing the present

____Increased connection ____Increased sense of personal validity

Describe how the skill helped or did not help you become more mindful: _____

_____

Describe the situation and how you practiced the skill:

_____

_____

_____

_____

Check if practicing this mindfulness skill has improved any of the following, *even a little bit*:

____Reduced suffering ____Increased happiness ____Increased ability to focus

____Decreased reactivity ____Increased wisdom ____Increased experiencing the present

____Increased connection ____Increased sense of personal validity

Describe how the skill helped or did not help you become more mindful: _____

_____

List any and all wise things you did this week: _____

Nonjudgmentalness, One-Mindfulness, Effectiveness Checklist

Due Date: _____   Name: _____ Week Starting: _____

Practice nonjudgmentalness: Check off an exercise each time you do one.

☐☐☐☐ 1. Say in your mind, "A judgmental thought arose in my mind."

☐☐☐☐ 2. Count judgmental thoughts.

☐☐☐☐ 3. Replace judgmental thoughts and statements with nonjudgmental thoughts and statements.

☐☐☐☐ 4. Observe your judgmental facial expressions, postures, voice tones.

☐☐☐☐ 5. Change judgmental expressions, postures, voice tones.

☐☐☐☐ 6. Stay very concrete and describe your day nonjudgmentally.

☐☐☐☐ 7. Write out a nonjudgmental description of an event that prompted an emotion.

☐☐☐☐ 8. Write out a nonjudgmental blow-by-blow account of a particularly important episode in your day.

☐☐☐☐ 9. Imagine a person you are angry with. Imagine understanding that person.

☐☐☐☐ 10. When you feel judgmental, practice half-smiling and/or willing hands.

Describe the situation and how you practiced nonjudgmentalness:

_____

_____

Practice one-mindfulness: Check off an exercise each time you do one.

☐☐☐☐ 11. Awareness while making tea or coffee.

☐☐☐☐ 12. Awareness while washing the dishes.

☐☐☐☐ 13. Awareness while hand-washing clothes.

☐☐☐☐ 14. Awareness while cleaning house.

☐☐☐☐ 15. Awareness while taking a slow-motion bath.

☐☐☐☐ 16. Awareness with meditation.

Describe the situation and how you practiced one-mindfulness:

_____

_____

Practice effectiveness: Check off an exercise each time you do one.

☐☐☐☐ 17. Give up being right

☐☐☐☐ 18. Drop willfulness

☐☐☐☐ 19. Doing what is effective

Describe the situation and how you practiced effectiveness:

_____

_____

List any and all wise things you did this week: _____

MINDFULNESS WORKSHEET 5B (Mindfulness Handouts 5–5c)

Nonjudgmentalness, One-Mindfulness, Effectiveness Calendar

Due Date: _____ Name: _____ Week Starting: _____

Check off at least two skills to practice this week: _____ Nonjudgmentally _____ One-mindfully _____ Effectively

While you are practicing skills, stay as aware and mindful as you can. Write it down later.

Name(s) of skill(s)	How did you practice the skill?	Describe your experience, including body sensations, emotions, and thoughts while practicing the skill	What is your experience now, after using the skill?
Example: *One-mindfully*	*I dusted my house and focused only on that task while doing it.*	*I experienced the softness of the cloth on my hands; I felt content I was able to do something useful; I started to think about all the other cleaning I needed to do afterward, but I brought my focus back to just doing the dusting.*	*I remember it felt good my husband noticed I cleaned up the house; I feel content I did my practice; I think I could have practiced better if my mind had drifted away less.*
Monday:			
Tuesday:			
Wednesday:			

(continued on next page)

Name(s) of skill(s)	How did you practice the skill?	Describe your experience, including body sensations, emotions, and thoughts while practicing the skill	What is your experience now, after using the skill?
Thursday:			
Friday:			
Saturday:			
Sunday:			

List any and all wise things you did this week: _____

Nonjudgmentalness Calendar

Due Date: _____   Name: _____   Week Starting: _____

Be aware of nonjudgmental thoughts and expressions when they happen. Use the following questions to focus your awareness on the details of the experience as it is happening. Write it down later.

Did you practice observing judgmental thoughts?	Did you count judgmental thoughts? If so, how many?	If you replaced a judgmental thought or assumption, what was the judgmental thought or assumption?	What was the replacement thought or assumption?	If you replaced judgmental with nonjudgmental facial or other physical expressions, please describe.	Describe any change after practicing.
Example: Yes	21	My boyfriend is such a jerk because he should have remembered to pick me up.	He did forget to pick me up! I wish he had not forgotten to pick me up.	I half-smiled and unclenched my fists.	
Monday:					
Tuesday:					
Wednesday:					

(continued on next page)

Did you practice observing judgmental thoughts?	Did you count judgmental thoughts? If so, how many?	If you replaced a judgmental thought or assumption, what was the judgmental thought or assumption?	What was the replacement thought or assumption.	If you replaced judgmental with nonjudgmental facial or other physical expressions, please describe.	Describe any change after practicing.
Thursday:					
Friday:					
Saturday:					
Sunday:					

List any and all wise things you did this week: _____

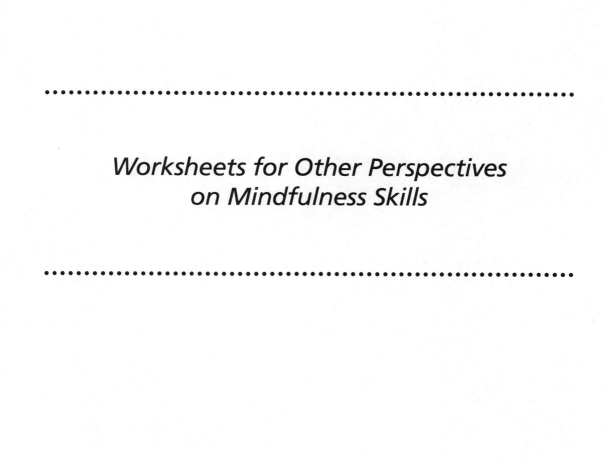

Worksheets for Other Perspectives on Mindfulness Skills

Loving Kindness

Due Date: _____ Name: _____ Week Starting: _____

Check off the types of loving kindness mindfulness practices you did this week. Write out descriptions of two different times when you practiced loving kindness. Use the back of this worksheet if more space is needed.

____To myself ____To a loved one ____To a friend ____To someone I was angry with
____To a difficult person ____To an enemy ____To all beings ____Other: _____

Describe the script you used (i.e., the warm wishes you sent):

1. _____
2. _____
3. _____
4. _____
5. _____

Check if practicing loving kindness has increased any of the following, *even a little bit* toward this person: ____Feelings of warmth or caring ____Love ____Compassion
____Feelings of connection ____Wisdom ____Happiness ____Sense of personal validity

Describe how the skill helped or did not help you become more compassionate: _____
_____

____To myself ____To a loved one ____To a friend ____To someone I was angry with
____To a difficult person ____To an enemy ____To all beings ____Other: _____

Describe the script you used (i.e., the warm wishes you sent): ____Same as above (check if correct).

1. _____
2. _____
3. _____
4. _____
5. _____

Check if practicing loving kindness has increased any of the following, *even a little bit* toward this person: ____Feelings of warmth or caring ____Love ____Compassion
____Feelings of connection ____Wisdom ____Happiness ____Sense of personal validity

Describe how the skill helped or did not help you become more compassionate: _____
_____

List any and all wise things you did this week: _____

Balancing Being Mind with Doing Mind

Due Date: _____ Name: _____ Week Starting: _____

Everyday Wise Mind practice: Check off Wise Mind practice exercises each time you do one.

☐☐☐☐ 1. Wrote out and then read an inspirational writing on mindfulness.

☐☐☐☐ 2. Set Wise Mind reminders to remind me to practice mindfulness.

☐☐☐☐ 3. Put written reminders to practice mindfulness in strategic places.

☐☐☐☐ 4. Made a deliberate effort to bring moment-to-moment awareness to an everyday activity.

☐☐☐☐ 5. Focused on just "this one moment" when I was overwhelmed, frazzled, or scattered.

☐☐☐☐ 6. Focused awareness on events in my everyday life.

☐☐☐☐ 7. Focused awareness on what needs to be done in my everyday life.

☐☐☐☐ 8. Acted willingly and did what was needed.

☐☐☐☐ 9. Did 3-minute Wise Mind to slow down "doing mind" in my everyday life.

☐☐☐☐ 10. Other (describe): _____

Describe one or more situations where you balanced being with doing mind:

_____

_____

How effective was the practice in helping you find Wise Mind in your everyday life?

Not effective: *I couldn't do the skill for even 1 minute. I got distracted or quit.*		*Somewhat effective:* *I was able to practice Wise Mind and became somewhat centered in my Wise Mind.*		*Very effective:* *I became centered in Wise Mind, and was free to do what needed to be done.*
1	**2**	**3**	**4**	**5**

Describe one or more situations where you balanced being with doing mind:

_____

_____

How effective was the practice in helping you find Wise Mind in your everyday life?

Not effective: *I couldn't do the skill for even 1 minute. I got distracted or quit.*		*Somewhat effective:* *I was able to practice Wise Mind and became somewhat centered in my Wise Mind.*		*Very effective:* *I became centered in Wise Mind, and was free to do what needed to be done.*
1	**2**	**3**	**4**	**5**

List any and all wise things you did this week: _____

_____

Mindfulness of Being and Doing Calendar

Due Date: _____   Name: _____   Week Starting: _____

Be aware of a moment when you feel frazzled, overwhelmed, or scattered at the time it is happening. Pay attention to your experience at that time. Try to bring your focus back to "just this one moment," not the next moment and not the past moment. Use the following questions to focus your awareness on the details of the experience as it is happening. Write it down later.

What was the experience?	What was the one activity in just one moment that you could bring your attention to?	How did your body feel doing one thing at a time?	Describe your experience of practicing the skill.	What is your experience now, after using the skill?
Example: Feeling overwhelmed at the number of dishes I had to wash before going to bed.	Washing just one dish.	Arms relaxed, hands felt warm and sudsy, back relaxed.	Relief, "Oh, only one dish," tension flowing out.	This was not so hard, but what about next time? I'll have to practice this.
Monday:				
Tuesday:				
Wednesday:				

(continued on next page)

What was the experience?	What was the one activity in just one moment that you could bring your attention to?	How did your body feel doing one thing at a time?	Describe your experience of practicing the skill.	What is your experience now, after using the skill?
Thursday:				
Friday:				
Saturday:				
Sunday:				

List any and all wise things you did this week: _____

Mindfulness of Pleasant Events Calendar

Due Date: _____   Name: _____   Week Starting: _____

Be aware of a pleasant event at the time it is happening. Pay attention to everyday, ordinary events that at the time feel pleasant to you. Try to experience the moment, even if it is only fleeting. Use the following questions to focus your awareness on the details of the experience as it is happening. Write it down later.

What was the experience?	What was the one activity in just one moment that you could bring your attention to?	How did your body feel during this experience?	Describe your emotions and thoughts while practicing the skill.	What is your experience now, after using the skill?
Example: *Seeing a bird while walking around green lake.*	*Yes.*	*Lightness across the face, aware of shoulders dropping, uplift of corners of mouth.*	*Relief, pleasure, "That's good," "How lovely (the bird) sings," "It's so nice to be outside."*	*It was such a small thing but I'm glad I noticed it.*
Monday:				
Tuesday:				
Wednesday:				

(continued on next page)

What was the experience?	What was the one activity in just one moment that you could bring your attention to?	How did your body feel during this experience?	Describe your emotions and thoughts while practicing the skill.	What is your experience now, after using the skill?
Thursday:				
Friday:				
Saturday:				
Sunday:				

List any and all wise things you did this week: _____

Mindfulness of Unpleasant Events Calendar

Due Date: _____ Name: _____ Week Starting: _____

Be aware of an unpleasant event at the time it is happening. Pay attention to everyday, ordinary events that at the time feel painful or unpleasant to you. Try to experience the moment, even if it is only fleeting. Use the following questions to focus your awareness on the details of the experience as it is happening. Write it down later.

What was the experience?	Were you aware of the unpleasant feelings *while* the event was happening?	How did your body feel during this experience?	Describe your emotions and thoughts while practicing the skill.	What is your experience now, after using the skill?
Example: *My boyfriend forgot my birthday.*	*Yes.*	*Tears just behind my eyes, sinking feeling in stomach, drooping of face and shoulders, tired.*	*Hurt, sadness, "He doesn't care enough to remember me," "Does he really love me?" Wanting to go to sleep until tomorrow.*	*He is a pretty forgetful guy. Maybe I need to remind him a lot.*
Monday:				
Tuesday:				
Wednesday:				

(continued on next page)

What was the experience?	Were you aware of the unpleasant feelings *while* the event was happening?	How did your body feel during this experience?	Describe your emotions and thoughts while practicing the skill.	What is your experience now, after using the skill?
Thursday:				
Friday:				
Saturday:				
Sunday:				

List any and all wise things you did this week: _____

Walking the Middle Path to Wise Mind

Due Date: _____ Name: _____ Week Starting: _____

WALKING THE MIDDLE PATH: Check off WISE MIND practice exercises each time you do one.

Worked at **balancing:**

☐☐☐☐ 1. Reasonable mind with emotion mind to get to Wise Mind.

☐☐☐☐ 2. Doing mind with being mind to get to Wise Mind.

☐☐☐☐ 3. Desire for change of the present moment with radical acceptance to get to Wise Mind.

☐☐☐☐ 4. Self-denial with self-indulgence to get to Wise Mind.

☐☐☐☐ 5. Other: _____

WALKING THE MIDDLE PATH: Describe one or more situations where you walked the middle path, and tell how you did this:

_____

_____

How effective was the practice in helping you walk the middle path?

Not effective: *I couldn't do the skill* *for even 1 minute. I got* *distracted or quit.*		*Somewhat effective:* *I was able to practice Wise Mind* *and became somewhat centered* *in my Wise Mind.*		*Very effective:* *I became centered in Wise* *Mind, and was free to do* *what needed to be done.*
1	**2**	**3**	**4**	**5**

WALKING THE MIDDLE PATH: Describe one or more situations where you walked the middle path, and tell how you did this:

_____

_____

How effective was the practice in helping you walk the middle path?

Not effective: *I couldn't do the skill* *for even 1 minute. I got* *distracted or quit.*		*Somewhat effective:* *I was able to practice Wise Mind* *and became somewhat centered* *in my Wise Mind.*		*Very effective:* *I became centered in Wise* *Mind, and was free to do* *what needed to be done.*
1	**2**	**3**	**4**	**5**

List any and all wise things you did this week: _____

Analyzing Yourself on the Middle Path

Due Date: _____   Name: _____ Week Starting: _____

1. **Figure out where you are off the middle path, toward one extreme or the other.** For each of the following Wise Mind dilemmas, put an X on the line that represents where you think you are most of the time. If you are fairly balanced, put the X in the middle. If you are out of balance, put the X near the end that you are too extreme on.

Reasonable mind	←——————————△——————————→	Emotion mind
Doing mind	←——————————△——————————→	Nothing-to-do mind
Intense desire for change of the moment	←——————————△——————————→	Radical acceptance of what is
Self-denial	←——————————△——————————→	Self-indulgence

2. **Choose one dilemma.** Describe *very specifically* what you are doing that is too much, and then describe what you do too little of.

Too much	Too little
_____	_____
_____	_____
_____	_____

3. **Check the facts.** Check for interpretations and opinions. Make sure that your list of activities you do too much of or too little of is in fact accurate. Check your own values in Wise Mind: Be sure to work on your middle path, not someone else's. Also check for **judgments.** Avoid "good," "bad," and judgmental language. Rewrite any items above if needed so that they are **factual and nonjudgmental.**

4. **Decide** on one (or at most two) *very specific* things to do in the next week to get closer to balance.

Do less	Do more
_____	_____
_____	_____
_____	_____

5. **Describe** what you did since last week: _____

6. **Rate** how effective the practice was in helping you become more balanced on the middle path. Rate it from 1 (did not help at all) to 5 (very effective, really helped): _____

List any and all wise things you did this week: _____

Walking the Middle Path Calendar

Due Date: _____   Name: _____   Week Starting: _____

Day	Describe the tension between the:		Describe in detail how you managed the tension between the pulls of the two sides.
	Pull to one side	**Pull to opposite side**	
Example: Doing projects around the house	Desperately working on lots of projects to renovate my house.	Watching TV, eating ice cream, leaving projects needed to sell house undone	I decided to do one small project each day and one medium project each week to improve the house. I also decided to have at least 1 hour each day of not thinking or worrying about the house, and instead doing something pleasant for myself.
Monday:			
Tuesday:			
Wednesday:			

(continued on next page)

Day	Describe the tension between the:		Describe in detail how you managed the tension between the pulls of the two sides.
	Pull to one side	Pull to opposite side	
Thursday:			
Friday:			
Saturday:			
Sunday:			

List any and all wise things you did this week: _____

INTERPERSONAL EFFECTIVENESS SKILLS

Introduction to Handouts and Worksheets

Interpersonal effectiveness skills help you build new relationships, strengthen current ones, and deal with conflict situations. They help you effectively ask for what you want and say no to unwanted requests. After a few handouts and worksheets for **Goals and Factors That Interfere**, three main groups of forms for interpersonal effectiveness skills are provided in DBT. The first set focuses on **Obtaining Objectives Skillfully**—that is, how to get what you want from others, while also maintaining your relationships and your self-respect. The second set, **Building Relationships and Ending Destructive Ones**, focuses on how to find friends, get them to like you, and maintain the relationships, as well as on how to end damaging relationships. The third set covers **Walking the Middle Path** skills, which in this module have to do with balancing acceptance and change in relationships.

Goals and Factors That Interfere

• **Interpersonal Effectiveness Handout 1: Goals of Interpersonal Effectiveness Skills.** This first handout overviews the goals for each of the three main sections of this module. The major overall goal is to be effective in getting what you want skillfully.

• **Interpersonal Effectiveness Worksheet 1: Pros and Cons of Using Interpersonal Skills.** Use this worksheet to decide whether to use interpersonal skills instead of power tactics or giving up and giving in to another person.

• **Interpersonal Effectiveness Handout 2: Factors in the Way of Interpersonal Effectiveness.** Lack of skills is only one factor that may prevent you from being effective with other people. This handout is helpful not only early in the module, but later in troubleshooting difficulties with using interpersonal effectiveness skills.

It can then be used with **Interpersonal Effectiveness Worksheet 7: Troubleshooting Interpersonal Effectiveness Skills,** and **Interpersonal Effectiveness Worksheet 9: Troubleshooting: When What You Are Doing Isn't Working.** These two worksheets cover the same topics, organized in the same sequence as Interpersonal Effectiveness Handout 2.

 • **Interpersonal Effectiveness Handout 2a: Myths in the Way of Interpersonal Effectiveness.** This handout can be useful if thoughts and beliefs get in the way of using interpersonal skills effectively. Use it with **Interpersonal Effectiveness Worksheet 2: Challenging Myths in the Way of Interpersonal Effectiveness.**

Obtaining Objectives Skillfully

 • **Interpersonal Effectiveness Handout 3: Overview: Obtaining Objectives Skillfully.** This handout overviews the skills covered in this section.

 • **Interpersonal Effectiveness Handout 4: Clarifying Goals in Interpersonal Situations.** Clarifying your goals is the first and most important interpersonal skill. It is the essential task of figuring out (1) what you actually want in any given situation and how important that is, compared to (2) keeping a positive relationship and (3) keeping your own self-respect. The skills you use depend on the relative importance of these three goals. Use this handout with **Interpersonal Effectiveness Worksheet 3: Figuring Out Goals in Interpersonal Situations.** In describing the "Prompting Event" on this worksheet, remember to use the mindfulness "what" skill of describing.

 • **Interpersonal Effectiveness Handout 5: Guidelines for Objectives Effectiveness: Getting What You Want (DEAR MAN).** This handout describes the skills for asking for something, saying no to another's request, and resisting pressure and maintaining your point of view. The skills are <u>D</u>escribe, <u>E</u>xpress, <u>A</u>ssert, <u>R</u>einforce; and (stay) <u>M</u>indful, <u>A</u>ppear confident, and <u>N</u>egotiate. You can use the term DEAR MAN to remember these. Two different worksheets can be used with this handout, as described next.

 • **Interpersonal Effectiveness Worksheet 4: Writing Out Interpersonal Effectiveness Scripts.** This worksheet is useful for figuring out what to say and do before practicing DEAR MAN skills. Notice also that the worksheet requires you to first write down your objectives, relationship, and self-respect goals. This worksheet can also be used for GIVE and FAST skills (see below).

 • **Interpersonal Effectiveness Worksheet 5: Tracking Interpersonal Effectiveness Skills Use.** This worksheet can be used to track your use of interpersonal skills. It asks you to figure out and write down your priorities and asks about conflicts in priorities. Finally, it asks you to record whether or not your objective was met, and what effect the interaction had on the relationship and your self-respect. This worksheet can be used with DEAR MAN, GIVE, and FAST skills.

 • **Interpersonal Effectiveness Handout 5a: Applying DEAR MAN Skills to a**

Difficult Current Interaction. This handout gives examples of how to handle situations where the other person also has very good interpersonal skills and refuses legitimate requests or keeps asking despite being told no. Use Interpersonal Effectiveness Worksheet 4, 5, or both with this handout (see above).

• **Interpersonal Effectiveness Handout 6: Guidelines for Relationship Effectiveness: Keeping the Relationship (GIVE).** Relationship effectiveness skills are aimed at maintaining or improving your relationship with the other person while you try to get what you want in the interaction. The term GIVE is a way to remember these skills. It stands for (be) Gentle, (act) Interested, Validate, and (use an) Easy manner. Use Interpersonal Effectiveness Worksheet 4, 5, or both with this handout.

• **Interpersonal Effectiveness Handout 6a: Expanding the V in GIVE: Levels of Validation.** This handout lists six different ways to validate. (See also Interpersonal Effectiveness Handouts 17 and 18, described later, for more on validation.) Interpersonal Effectiveness Worksheets 4 and 5 can be used with this handout.

• **Interpersonal Effectiveness Handout 7: Guidelines for Self-Respect Effectiveness: Keeping Respect for Yourself (FAST).** Self-respect effectiveness skills help you to keep or improve your self-respect while you try to get what you want in an interaction. The term FAST is a way to remember these skills: (be) Fair, (no) Apologies, Stick to values, and (be) Truthful. Interpersonal Effectiveness Worksheets 4 and 5 can be used with this handout.

• **Interpersonal Effectiveness Handout 8: Evaluating Options for Whether or How Intensely to Ask for Something or Say No.** Before asking for something or saying no to another, consider how intensely to ask or say no—and whether to ask or say no at all. This handout lists the factors to consider in making a decision. Use **Interpersonal Effectiveness Worksheet 6: The Dime Game: Figuring Out How Strongly to Ask or Say No** with this handout to figure out your best option in a particular situation.

• **Interpersonal Effectiveness Handout 9: Troubleshooting: When What You Are Doing Isn't Working.** Difficulty in obtaining an objective can be due to many possible factors. When you can identify the problem, you can often solve it and be more effective in getting what you want. This handout provides questions for diagnosing which factors are reducing your interpersonal effectiveness. Use **Interpersonal Effectiveness Worksheet 7: Troubleshooting Interpersonal Effectiveness Skills** with this handout.

Building Relationships and Ending Destructive Ones

• **Interpersonal Effectiveness Handout 10: Overview: Building Relationships and Ending Destructive Ones.** This handout briefly overviews the skills taught in this section of the module.

• **Interpersonal Effectiveness Handout 11: Finding and Getting People to Like You.** Finding potential friends and getting them to like you often both require an active effort. The handout summarizes where to look and how to look. Record your practice efforts for this on **Interpersonal Effectiveness Worksheet 8: Finding and Getting People to Like You.**

• **Interpersonal Effectiveness Handout 11a: Identifying Skills to Find People and Get Them to Like You.** This is a quick multiple-choice quiz on the information in Interpersonal Effectiveness Handout 11.

• **Interpersonal Effectiveness Handout 12: Mindfulness of Others.** Friendships are easier to form and last longer when we remember to be mindful of the other person. Notice that the three mindfulness skills described on this handout are the three core mindfulness "what" skills (observing, describing, and participating) taught in the Mindfulness module. Use **Interpersonal Effectiveness Worksheet 9: Mindfulness of Others** to record practice of this skill.

• **Interpersonal Effectiveness Handout 12a: Identifying Mindfulness of Others.** This is a brief multiple-choice quiz on the skill of mindfulness of others.

• **Interpersonal Effectiveness Handout 13: Ending Relationships.** The skills for ending relationships described on this handout are drawn from the Mindfulness (Wise Mind), Emotion Regulation (problem solving, coping ahead, opposite action), and Interpersonal Effectiveness (DEAR MAN, GIVE FAST) skills modules. The one new skill is practicing safety first when ending abusive or life-threatening relationships. If you are thinking about ending a relationship, use **Interpersonal Effectiveness Worksheet 10: Ending Relationships** to weigh the factors and plan for use of these skills. If trying to leave an abusive or dangerous relationship, call a domestic violence hotline number first (either a local number or the national number listed on the worksheet). Interpersonal Effectiveness Worksheet 1: Pros and Cons of Using Interpersonal Skills may also be useful with this handout.

• **Interpersonal Effectiveness Handout 13a: Identifying How to End Relationships.** This is a brief multiple-choice quiz on how to end relationships.

Walking the Middle Path

• **Interpersonal Effectiveness Handout 14: Overview: Walking the Middle Path.** This handout briefly overviews the skills in this section: dialectics, validation, and behavior change strategies. These skills help you to effectively manage yourself and your relationships.

• **Interpersonal Effectiveness Handout 15: Dialectics.** A dialectical stance is essential for walking a middle path and for decreasing a sense of isolation, conflict, and polarities. This handout outlines the basics of a dialectical perspective.

• **Interpersonal Effectiveness Handout 16: How to Think and Act Dialectically.** This is an extension of Interpersonal Effectiveness Handout 15 and gives examples of how to think and act dialectically. There are three worksheets with different formats for recording dialectics practice, described next.

• **Interpersonal Effectiveness Worksheet 11: Practicing Dialectics, Interpersonal Effectiveness Worksheet 11a: Dialectics Checklist,** and **Interpersonal Effectiveness Worksheet 11b: Noticing When You're Not Dialectical,** can be used with Interpersonal Effectiveness Handout 16. Worksheet 11 provides space for recording two practices over the week. Worksheet 11a provides for multiple practices of multiple skills. Worksheet 11b is intended to help raise awareness of opportunities to be dialectical and of the consequences when not being dialectical.

• **Interpersonal Effectiveness Handout 16a: Examples of Opposite Sides That Can Both Be True.** Dialectics tells us that the universe is filled with opposing sides, and that two things that seem like opposites can both be true. This handout lists examples of opposites that can both be true.

• **Interpersonal Effectiveness Handout 16b: Important Opposites to Balance.** This handout lists opposite aspects of life and living that are important to keep in balance.

• **Interpersonal Effectiveness Handout 16c: Identifying Dialectics.** This handout is a brief multiple-choice quiz. It asks you to check the most dialectical responses.

• **Interpersonal Effectiveness Handout 17: Validation.** Validation of others' feelings, beliefs, experiences, and actions is essential in building any relationship of trust and intimacy. This handout reviews what validation is, what is most important to validate, and key points to remember about validation.

• **Interpersonal Effectiveness Handout 18: A "How To" Guide to Validation.** This handout lists the six levels of validation and gives examples of each. Fill out **Interpersonal Effectiveness Worksheet 12: Validating Others** whenever you have an opportunity to practice validation skills, whether or not you actually practiced the skills.

• **Interpersonal Effectiveness Handout 18a: Identifying Validation.** This handout is a brief multiple-choice quiz on validation.

• **Interpersonal Effectiveness Handout 19: Recovering from Invalidation.** Invalidation can be helpful or harmful. Either way, it usually hurts. This handout lists how to respond effectively when you are invalidated by someone. Fill out **Interpersonal Effectiveness Worksheet 13: Self-Validation and Self-Respect** whenever you have an opportunity to practice self-validation skills whether or not you actually practiced them.

• **Interpersonal Effectiveness Handout 19a: Identifying Self-Validation.** This is a brief multiple-choice quiz on responding to invalidation.

• **Interpersonal Effectiveness Handout 20: Strategies for Increasing the Probability of Desired Behaviors.** This handout describes very effective strategies for increasing behaviors you want in yourself or others: behavior reinforcement and new behavior shaping. To be effective in changing behaviors, learn these strategies and put them into action. To record your practice, use **Interpersonal Effectiveness Worksheet 14: Changing Behavior with Reinforcement.**

• **Interpersonal Effectiveness Handout 21: Strategies for Decreasing or Stopping Undesired Behaviors.** This handout describes effective strategies for decreasing or stopping unwanted behaviors—extinction, satiating, and punishment. To record your practice, use **Interpersonal Effectiveness Worksheet 15: Changing Behavior by Extinguishing or Punishing It.**

• **Interpersonal Effectiveness Handout 22: Tips for Using Behavior Change Strategies Effectively.** Reinforcement, extinction, and punishment each involve different kinds of consequences. This handout outlines important issues in selecting and implementing consequences.

• **Interpersonal Effectiveness Handout 22a: Identifying Effective Behavior Change Strategies.** This is a brief multiple-choice quiz on behavior change strategies.

Interpersonal Effectiveness Handouts

Handouts for Goals and Factors That Interfere

Goals of Interpersonal Effectiveness

BE SKILLFUL IN GETTING WHAT YOU WANT AND NEED FROM OTHERS

❑ Get others to do things you would like them to do.

❑ Get others to take your opinions seriously.

❑ Say no to unwanted requests effectively.

❑ Other: _____

BUILD RELATIONSHIPS AND END DESTRUCTIVE ONES

❑ Strengthen current relationships.

    ❑ Don't let hurts and problems build up.

    ❑ Use relationship skills to head off problems.

    ❑ Repair relationships when needed.

    ❑ Resolve conflicts before they get overwhelming.

❑ Find and build new relationships.

❑ End hopeless relationships.

❑ Other: _____

WALK THE MIDDLE PATH

❑ Create and maintain balance in relationships.

❑ Balance acceptance and change in relationships.

❑ Other: _____

Factors in the Way of Interpersonal Effectiveness

☐ **YOU DON'T HAVE THE INTERPERSONAL SKILLS YOU NEED**

YOU DON'T KNOW WHAT YOU WANT

☐ You have the skills, but can't decide what you really want from the other person.

☐ You can't figure out how to balance your needs versus the other person's needs:
  ☐ Asking for too much versus not asking for anything.
  ☐ Saying no to everything versus giving in to everything.

YOUR EMOTIONS ARE GETTING IN THE WAY

☐ You have the skills, but emotions (anger, pride, contempt, fear, shame, guilt) control what you do.

YOU FORGET YOUR LONG-TERM GOALS FOR SHORT-TERM GOALS

☐ You put your immediate urges and wants ahead of your long-term goals. The future vanishes from your mind.

OTHER PEOPLE ARE GETTING IN YOUR WAY

☐ You have the skills but other people get in the way.

☐ Other people are more powerful than you.

☐ Other people may be threatened or may not like you if you get what you want.

☐ Other people may not do what you want unless you sacrifice your self-respect, at least a little.

YOUR THOUGHTS AND BELIEFS ARE GETTING IN THE WAY

☐ Worries about negative consequences if you ask for what you want or say no to someone's request get in the way of acting effectively.

☐ Beliefs that you don't deserve what you want stop you in your tracks.

☐ Beliefs that others don't deserve what they want make you ineffective.

Myths in the Way of Interpersonal Effectiveness

Myths in the Way of Objectives Effectiveness

☐ 1. I don't deserve to get what I want or need.

☐ 2. If I make a request, this will show that I am a very weak person.

☐ 3. I have to know whether a person is going to say yes before I make a request.

☐ 4. If I ask for something or say no, I can't stand it if someone gets upset with me.

☐ 5. If they say no, it will kill me.

☐ 6. Making requests is a really pushy (bad, self-centered, selfish, etc.) thing to do.

☐ 7. Saying no to a request is always a selfish thing to do.

☐ 8. I should be willing to sacrifice my own needs for others.

☐ 9. I must be really inadequate if I can't fix this myself.

☐ 10. Obviously, the problem is just in my head. If I would just think differently I wouldn't have to bother everybody else.

☐ 11. If I don't have what I want or need, it doesn't make any difference; I don't care really.

☐ 12. Skillfulness is a sign of weakness.

Other myth: _____

Other myth: _____

Myths in the Way of Relationship and Self-Respect Effectiveness

☐ 13. I shouldn't have to ask (say no); they should know what I want (and do it).

☐ 14. They should have known that their behavior would hurt my feelings; I shouldn't have to tell them.

☐ 15. I shouldn't have to negotiate or work at getting what I want.

☐ 16. Other people should be willing to do more for my needs.

☐ 17. Other people should like, approve of, and support me.

☐ 18. They don't deserve my being skillful or treating them well.

☐ 19. Getting what I want when I want it is most important.

☐ 20. I shouldn't be fair, kind, courteous, or respectful if others are not so toward me.

☐ 21. Revenge will feel so good; it will be worth any negative consequences.

☐ 22. Only wimps have values.

☐ 23. Everybody lies.

☐ 24. Getting what I want is more important than how I get it; the ends really do justify the means.

Other myth: _____

Other myth: _____

*Handouts for Obtaining
Objectives Skillfully*

Overview:
Obtaining Objectives Skillfully

CLARIFYING PRIORITIES

How important is:

Getting what you want/obtaining your goal?

Keeping the relationship?

Maintaining your self-respect?

OBJECTIVES EFFECTIVENESS: DEAR MAN

Be effective in asserting your rights and wishes.

RELATIONSHIP EFFECTIVENESS: GIVE

Act in such a way that you maintain positive relationships and that others feel good about themselves and about you.

SELF-RESPECT EFFECTIVENESS: FAST

Act in such a way that you keep your self-respect.

FACTORS TO CONSIDER

Decide how firm or intense you want to be in asking for something or saying no.

Clarifying Goals in Interpersonal Situations

OBJECTIVES EFFECTIVENESS: Getting What You Want from Another Person

- Obtaining your legitimate rights.
- Getting another person to do something you want that person to do.
- Saying no to an unwanted or unreasonable request.
- Resolving an interpersonal conflict.
- Getting your opinion or point of view taken seriously.

Questions

1. *What specific **results or changes** do I want from this interaction?*
2. *What do I have to do to get the results? What will work?*

RELATIONSHIP EFFECTIVENESS: Keeping and Improving the Relationship

- Acting in such a way that the other person keeps liking and respecting you.
- Balancing immediate goals with the good of the long-term relationship.
- Maintaining relationships that matter to you.

Questions

1. *How do I want the **other person to feel about me** after the interaction is over (whether or not I get the results or changes I want)?*
2. *What do I have to do to get (or keep) this relationship?*

SELF-RESPECT EFFECTIVENESS: Keeping or Improving Self-Respect

- Respecting your own values and beliefs.
- Acting in a way that makes you feel moral.
- Acting in a way that makes you feel capable and effective.

Questions

1. *How do I want to **feel about myself** after the interaction is over (whether or not I get the results or changes I want)?*
2. *What do I have to do to feel that way about myself? What will work?*

Guidelines for Objectives Effectiveness:
Getting What You Want (DEAR MAN)

A way to remember these skills is to remember the term **DEAR MAN:**

> **D**escribe
> **E**xpress
> **A**ssert
> **R**einforce
> (Stay) **M**indful
> **A**ppear Confident
> **N**egotiate

Describe

Describe the current SITUATION (if necessary). Stick to the facts.
Tell the person exactly what you are reacting to.

"You told me you would be home by dinner but you didn't get here until 11."

Express

Express your FEELINGS and OPINIONS about the situation.
Don't assume that the other person knows how you feel.

"When you come home so late, I start worrying about you."

Use phrases such as *"I want"* instead of *"You should," "I don't want"* instead of *"You shouldn't."*

Assert

Assert yourself by ASKING for what you want or SAYING NO clearly.
Do not assume that others will figure out what you want.
Remember that others cannot read your mind.

"I would really like it if you would call me when you are going to be late."

Reinforce

Reinforce (reward) the person ahead of time (so to speak)
by explaining positive effects of getting what you want or need.
If necessary, also clarify the negative consequences of not getting what you want or need.

"I would be so relieved, and a lot easier to live with, if you do that."

Remember also to reward desired behavior after the fact.

(*continued on next page*)

(Stay)

Mindful

Keep your focus ON YOUR GOALS.
Maintain your position. Don't be distracted. Don't get off the topic.

"Broken record": Keep asking, saying no, or expressing your opinion over and over and over.
Just keep replaying the same thing again and again.

Ignore attacks: If another person attacks, threatens, or tries to change the subject,
ignore the threats, comments, or attempts to divert you.
Do not respond to attacks. Ignore distractions.
Just keep making your point.

"I would still like a call."

Appear confident

Appear EFFECTIVE and competent.

Use a confident voice tone and physical manner;
make good eye contact.

No stammering, whispering, staring at the floor, retreating.

No saying, "I'm not sure," etc.

Negotiate

Be willing to GIVE TO GET.
Offer and ask for other solutions to the problem.
Reduce your request.
Say no, but offer to do something else or to solve the problem another way.
Focus on what will work.

"How about if you text me when you think you might be late?"

Turn the tables: Turn the problem over to the other person.
Ask for other solutions.

"What do you think we should do? . . . I can't just stop worrying about
you [or I'm not willing to]."

Other ideas: _____

_____

_____

_____

_____

_____

_____

_____

_____

Applying DEAR MAN Skills
to a Difficult Current Interaction

To turn around really difficult situations, focus the skills on the other person's behavior right now.

When other people have really good skills themselves, and keep refusing your legitimate requests or pestering you to do something you don't want to do.

Apply DEAR MAN Skills

1. **Describe the current interaction.** If the "broken record" and ignoring don't work, make a statement about what is happening between you and the person now, *but without imputing motives.*

   Example: "You keep asking me over and over, even though I have already said no several times," or "It is hard to keep asking you to empty the dishwasher when it is your month to do it."

   Not: "You obviously don't want to hear what I am saying," "You obviously don't care about me," "Well, it's obvious that what I have to say doesn't matter to you," "Obviously you think I'm stupid."

2. **Express feelings or opinions about the interaction.** For instance, in the middle of an interaction that is not going well, you can express your feelings of discomfort in the situation.

   Example: "I am sorry I cannot do what you want, but I'm finding it hard to keep discussing it," or "It's becoming very uncomfortable for me to keep talking about this, since I can't help it. I am starting to feel angry about it," or "I'm not sure you think this is important for you to do."

   Not: "I hate you!", "Every time we talk about this, you get defensive," "Stop patronizing me!"

3. **Assert wishes in the situation.** When another person is pestering you, you can ask him or her to stop it. When a person is refusing a request, you can suggest that you put the conversation off until another time. Give the other person a chance to think about it.

   Example: "Please don't ask me again. My answer won't change," or "OK, let's stop discussing this now and pick it up again sometime tomorrow," or "Let's cool down for a while and then get together to figure out a solution."

   Not: "Would you shut up?" "You should do this!", "You should really calm down and do what's right here."

4. **Reinforce.** When you are saying no to someone who keeps asking, or when someone won't take your opinion seriously, suggest ending the conversation, since you aren't going to change your mind anyway. When trying to get someone to do something for you, you can suggest that you will come up with a better offer later.

   Example: "Let's stop talking about this now. I'm not going to change my mind, and I think this is just going to get frustrating for both of us," or "OK, I can see you don't want to do this, so let's see if we can come up with something that will make you more willing to do it."

   Not: "If you don't do this for me, I'll never do anything for you ever again," "If you keep asking me, I'll get a restraining order against you," "Gosh, you must be a terrible person for not doing this/for asking me to do this."

Guidelines for Relationship Effectiveness: Keeping the Relationship (GIVE)

A way to remember these skills is to remember the word **GIVE (DEAR MAN, GIVE):**

(Be) **G**entle
(Act) **I**nterested
Validate
(Use an) **E**asy manner

(Be)
Gentle | BE NICE and respectful.

No attacks: | No verbal or physical attacks. No hitting, clenching fists. No harassment of any kind. Express anger directly with words.

No threats: | If you have to describe painful consequences for not getting what you want, describe them calmly and without exaggerating.
No "manipulative" statements, no hidden threats. No "I'll kill myself if you . . . "
Tolerate a "no." Stay in the discussion even if it gets painful. Exit gracefully.

No judging: | No moralizing. No "If you were a good person, you would . . . "
No "You should . . . " or "You shouldn't . . . " Abandon blame.

No sneering: | No smirking, eye rolling, sucking teeth. No cutting off or walking away.
No saying, "That's stupid, don't be sad," "I don't care what you say."

(Act)
Interested | LISTEN and APPEAR INTERESTED in the other person.
Listen to the other person's point of view.
Face the person; maintain eye contact; lean toward the person rather than away. Don't interrupt or talk over the person.
Be sensitive to the person's wish to have the discussion at a later time. Be patient.

Validate | With WORDS AND ACTIONS, show that you understand the other person's feelings and thoughts about the situation. See the world from the other person's point of view, and then say or act on what you see.

"I realize this is hard for you, and . . . ", "I see that you are busy, and . . . "

Go to a private place when the person is uncomfortable talking in a public place.

(Use an)
Easy manner | Use a little humor.
SMILE. Ease the person along. Be light-hearted. Sweet-talk.
Use a "soft sell" over a "hard sell." Be "political."
Leave your attitude at the door.

Other ideas: _____

_____

_____

Expanding the V in GIVE: Levels of Validation

1. ❑ **Pay Attention:** Look interested in the other person instead of bored (no multitasking).

2. ❑ **Reflect Back:** Say back what you heard the other person say or do, to be sure you understand exactly what the person is saying. No judgmental language or tone of voice!

3. ❑ **"Read Minds":** Be sensitive to what is *not* being said by the other person. Pay attention to facial expressions, body language, what is happening, and what you know about the person already. Show you understand in words or by your actions. Check it out and make sure you are right. Let go if you are not.

4. ❑ **Understand:** Look for how what the other person is feeling, thinking, or doing makes sense, based on the person's past experiences, present situation, and/or current state of mind or physical condition (i.e., the causes).

5. ❑ **Acknowledge the Valid:** Look for how the person's feelings, thinking, or actions are valid responses because they fit current facts, or are understandable because they are a logical response to current facts.

6. ❑ **Show Equality:** Be yourself! Don't "one-up" or "one-down" the other person. Treat the other as an equal, not as fragile or incompetent.

Guidelines for Self-Respect Effectiveness: Keeping Respect for Yourself (FAST)

A way to remember these skills is to remember the word **FAST (DEAR MAN, GIVE FAST).**

(Be) <u>F</u>air
(No) <u>A</u>pologies
<u>S</u>tick to Values
(Be) <u>T</u>ruthful

(Be) Fair

Be fair to YOURSELF and to the OTHER person.
Remember to VALIDATE YOUR OWN feelings and wishes,
as well as the other person's.

(No) Apologies

Don't overapologize.
No apologizing for being alive or for making a request at all.
No apologies for having an opinion, for disagreeing.
No LOOKING ASHAMED, with eyes and head down or body slumped.
No invalidating the valid.

Stick to values

Stick to YOUR OWN values.
Don't sell out your values or integrity for reasons that aren't VERY important.
Be clear on what you believe is the moral or valued way of thinking and
acting, and "stick to your guns."

(Be) Truthful

Don't lie. Don't act helpless when you are not.
Don't exaggerate or make up excuses.

Other ideas: _____

_____

_____

_____

_____

_____

Evaluating Options for Whether or How Intensely to Ask for Something or Say No

Before asking for something or saying no to a request, you have to decide how intensely you want to hold your ground.

Options range from **very low** intensity, where you are very flexible and accept the situation as it is, to **very high** intensity, where you try every skill you know to change the situation and get what you want.

OPTIONS

Low intensity (let go, give in)

Asking		Saying No
Don't ask; don't hint.	1	Do what the other person wants without being asked.
Hint indirectly; take no.	2	Don't complain; do it cheerfully.
Hint openly; take no.	3	Do it, even if you're not cheerful about it.
Ask tentatively; take no.	4	Do it, but show that you'd rather not.
Ask gracefully, but take no.	5	Say you'd rather not, but do it gracefully.
Ask confidently; take no.	6	Say no confidently, but reconsider.
Ask confidently; resist no.	7	Say no confidently; resist saying yes.
Ask firmly; resist no.	8	Say no firmly; resist saying yes.
Ask firmly; insist; negotiate; keep trying.	9	Say no firmly; resist; negotiate; keep trying.
Ask and don't take no for an answer.	10	**Don't do it.**

High intensity (stay firm)

(*continued on next page*)

FACTORS TO CONSIDER

> **When deciding how firm or intense
> you want to be in asking or saying no, think about:**
>
> 1. The other person's or your own **capability.**
>
> 2. Your **priorities.**
>
> 3. The effect of your actions on your **self-respect.**
>
> 4. Your or the other's moral and legal **rights** in the situation.
>
> 5. Your **authority** over the person (or his or hers over you).
>
> 6. The type of **relationship** you have with the person.
>
> 7. The effect of your action on **long- versus short-term goals.**
>
> 8. The degree of **give and take** in your relationship.
>
> 9. Whether you have done your **homework** to prepare.
>
> 10. The **timing** of your request or refusal.

1. CAPABILITY:
- Is the person able to give you what you want? If YES, raise the intensity of ASKING.
- Do you have what the person wants? If NO, raise the intensity of NO.

2. PRIORITIES:
- Are your GOALS very important? Increase intensity.
- Is your RELATIONSHIP shaky? Consider reducing intensity.
- Is your SELF-RESPECT on the line? Intensity should fit your values.

3. SELF-RESPECT:
- Do you usually do things for yourself? Are you careful to avoid acting helpless when you are not? If YES, raise the intensity of ASKING.
- Will saying no make you feel bad about yourself, even when you are thinking about it wisely? If NO, raise the intensity of NO.

4. RIGHTS:
- Is the person required by law or moral code to give you what you want? If YES, raise the intensity of ASKING.
- Are you required to give the person what he or she is asking for? Would saying no violate the other person's rights? If NO, raise the intensity of NO.

5. AUTHORITY:
- Are you responsible for directing the person or telling the person what to do? If YES, raise the intensity of ASKING.
- Does the person have authority over you (e.g., your boss, your teacher)? And is what the person is asking within his or her authority? If NO, raise the intensity of NO.

(continued on next page)

6. **RELATIONSHIP:**
   - Is what you want appropriate to the current relationship? If YES, raise the intensity of ASKING.
   - Is what the person is asking for appropriate to your current relationship? If NO, raise the intensity of NO.

7. **LONG-TERM VERSUS SHORT-TERM GOALS:**
   - Will not asking for what you want keep the peace now but create problems in the long run? If YES, raise the intensity of ASKING.
   - Is giving in to keep the peace right now more important than the long-term welfare of the relationship? Will you eventually regret or resent saying no? If NO, raise the intensity of NO.

8. **GIVE AND TAKE:**
   - What have you done for the person? Are you giving at least as much as you ask for? Are you willing to give if the person says yes? If YES, raise the intensity of ASKING.
   - Do you owe this person a favor? Does he or she do a lot for you? If NO, raise the intensity of NO.

9. **HOMEWORK:**
   - Have you done your homework? Do you know all the facts you need to know to support your request? Are you clear about what you want? If YES, raise the intensity of ASKING.
   - Is the other person's request clear? Do you know what you are agreeing to? If NO, raise the intensity of NO.

10. **TIMING:**
    - Is this a good time to ask? Is the person "in the mood" for listening and paying attention to you? Are you catching the person when he or she is likely to say yes to your request? If YES, raise the intensity of ASKING.
    - Is this a bad time to say no? Should you hold off answering for a while? If NO, raise the intensity of NO.

Other factors: _____

_____

_____

_____

_____

Troubleshooting:
When What You Are Doing Isn't Working

1

Do I have the skills I need? Check out the instructions.

Review what has already been tried.

- Do I know how to be skillful in getting what I want?
- Do I know how to say what I want to say?
- Do I follow the skill instructions to the letter?

2

Do I know what I really want in this interaction?

Ask:

- Am I undecided about what I really want in this interaction?
- Am I unsure of my priorities?
- Am I having trouble balancing:
  - Asking for too much versus too little?
  - Saying no to everything versus saying yes to everything?
- Is fear or shame getting in the way of knowing what I really want?

3

Are short-term goals getting in the way of long-term goals?

Ask:

- Is "NOW, NOW, NOW" winning out over getting what I really want in the future?
- Is emotion mind controlling what I say and do instead of WISE MIND?

(continued on next page)

4

Are my emotions getting in the way of using my skills?

Ask:

- Do I get too upset to use my skills?
- Are my emotions so HIGH that I am over my skills breakdown point?

5

Are worries, assumptions, and myths getting in my way?

Ask:

- Are THOUGHTS about bad consequences blocking my action?
  "They won't like me," "She will think I am stupid."
- Are THOUGHTS about not deserving things getting in my way?
  "I am such a bad person I don't deserve this."
- Am I calling myself NAMES that stop me from doing anything?
  "I won't do it right," "I'll probably fall apart," "I'm so stupid."
- Do I believe MYTHS about interpersonal effectiveness?
  "If I make a request, this will show that I am a weak person,"
  "Only wimps have values."

6

Is the environment more powerful than my skills?

Ask:

- Are the people who have what I want or need more powerful than I am?
- Are other people more in control of the situation than I am?
- Will others be threatened if I get what I want?
- Do others have reasons for not liking me if I get what I want?

7

Other ideas:

*Handouts for Building Relationships
and Ending Destructive Ones*

Overview:
Building Relationships
and Ending Destructive Ones

FINDING AND GETTING PEOPLE TO LIKE YOU

Proximity, similarity, conversation skills,
expressing liking, and joining groups

MINDFULNESS OF OTHERS

Building closeness through mindfulness of others

ENDING DESTRUCTIVE/
INTERFERING RELATIONSHIPS

Staying in WISE MIND

Using skills

Staying safe

Finding and Getting People to Like You

REMEMBER: <u>ALL</u> HUMAN BEINGS ARE LOVABLE.

But finding friends may take effort on your part.

LOOK FOR PEOPLE WHO ARE CLOSE BY YOU.

Familiarity often leads to liking and sometimes love.

To find people you might like and who might like you, it is important to make sure that you are frequently around and visible to a group of people. Many people find friends who are classmates or members of groups they join, or who work at or go to the same places.

LOOK FOR PEOPLE WHO ARE SIMILAR TO YOU.

We often make friends with people who share our interests and attitudes.

Though always agreeing with someone will not make you more attractive to them, a lot of people are attracted to those who share the same important interests and attitudes, such as politics, lifestyle, morals.

WORK ON YOUR CONVERSATION SKILLS.

Ask and respond to questions; respond with a little more info than requested.

Make small talk; don't underestimate the value of chit-chat.

Self-disclose skillfully; keep your self-disclosure close to that of the other person.

Don't interrupt; don't start talking just fractionally before or after someone else.

Learn things to talk about: Watch others; read; increase your activities and experiences.

EXPRESS LIKING (SELECTIVELY).

We often like the people we think like us.

Express genuine liking for the other person. But don't try to suck up to the other person or grovel. Find things to compliment that are not super-obvious. Don't praise too much too often, and never use compliments to obtain favors.

*(**continued on next page**)*

JOIN AN ONGOING GROUP CONVERSATION.

If we wait for people to approach us, we may never have friends.

Sometimes we must make the first move in finding friends. This often requires us to know how to tell if a group is open or closed, and then, when it is open, how to approach and join in the ongoing group.

FIGURE OUT IF A GROUP IS OPEN OR CLOSED.

In open groups new members are welcome.

In closed groups new members may not be welcome.

Open Groups	Closed Groups
• Everyone is standing somewhat apart. • Members occasionally glance around the room. • There are gaps in the conversation. • Members are talking about a topic of general interest.	• Everyone is standing close together. • Members attend exclusively to each other. • There is a very animated conversation with few gaps. • Members seem to be pairing off.

FIGURE OUT HOW TO JOIN AN OPEN GROUP CONVERSATION.

Ways of Joining an Open Group	Potential Outcomes
Move gradually closer to the group.	It may not be clear from the slowness of your approach that you want to join them; it might even look as though you were creeping up and trying to eavesdrop!
Offer to refill members' glasses/serve them food.	That could be overdoing things a bit. What would you do if they refused more food/drinks? Would it be clear enough that you wanted to join the group?
Stand beside them and chip in on their conversation.	That might seem rude. They haven't invited you to join them, and anyway, what exactly are you going to say when you chip in?
Go up and introduce yourself.	Isn't that overly formal? Having introduced yourself, then what do you say? Will they introduce themselves to you? Wouldn't you interrupt the conversation?
Wait for a break in the conversation, stand beside a friendly-looking member of the group and say something like "Mind if I join you?"	**This makes your intention clear and doesn't seem rude or interrupt the conversation; group members can then choose whether to introduce themselves or not.**

Identifying Skills to Find People
and Get Them to Like You

For each A and B pair, check the more effective responses.

☐ **1A.** Realize that good relationships depend on what you do.
☐ **1B.** Think of relationships in vague, abstract terms.

☐ **7A.** Stay out of conversations other people are having, so people know you're respectful.
☐ **7B.** Politely ask to join in conversations, so you can meet more people.

☐ **2A.** Expect people to beat a path to your door.
☐ **2B.** Create and make full use of opportunities to come into regular contact with others.

☐ **8A.** Say nothing or everything about yourself, regardless of what others reveal.
☐ **8B.** Disclose roughly the same amount of personal information to others as they disclose to you.

☐ **3A.** Mix with people who share your attitudes and interests.
☐ **3B.** Mix with people with whom you have little in common.

☐ **9A.** Keep good opinions of others to yourself.
☐ **9B.** If you like others, let them know.

☐ **4A.** Mix with people who respond positively to you and to life generally.
☐ **4B.** Mix with cynics and pessimists.

☐ **10A.** Protect yourself, and comment only on good points that are obvious to anyone and everyone.
☐ **10B.** Don't express liking indiscriminately.

☐ **5A.** Express your opinions and attitudes, so that others can recognize similarities with you.
☐ **5B.** Keep your opinions and attitudes to yourself.

☐ **11A.** Rely on flattery to get what you want when you think it will work.
☐ **11B.** Don't use flattery to influence others.

☐ **6A.** Answer questions briefly, and seldom ask or return them.
☐ **6B.** Show interest in others by asking questions.

☐ **12A.** Stand near a friendly-looking person in a new group, wait for a lull in the conversation, and then ask if it's OK for you to join the group.
☐ **12B.** Stand near a group of new people and make sure your comments or opinions are heard.

Mindfulness of Others

FRIENDSHIPS LAST LONGER WHEN WE ARE MINDFUL.

OBSERVE

❑ Pay attention with interest and curiosity to others around you.
❑ Stop multitasking; focus on the people you are with.
❑ Stay in the present rather than planning what to say next.
❑ Let go of a focus on self, and focus on others around you.
❑ Be open to new information about others.
❑ Notice judgmental thoughts about others, and let them go.
❑ Give up clinging to always being right.

DESCRIBE

❑ Replace judgmental words with descriptive words.
❑ Avoid assuming or interpreting what other people think about you without checking the facts. (Remember, *no one* has ever observed another person's thoughts, motives, intentions, feelings, emotions, desires, or experiences.)
❑ Avoid questioning other people's motives (unless you have very good reasons to do so).
❑ Give others the benefit of the doubt.

PARTICIPATE

❑ Throw yourself into interactions with others.
❑ Go with the flow, rather than trying to control the flow.
❑ Become one with group activities and conversations.

Identifying Mindfulness of Others

For each A and B pair, check the more effective response.

- ❑ **1A.** Multi-task and expect the other person to understand.
- ❑ **1B.** Give your complete attention to the person you are with.

- ❑ **2A.** Figure that if you already know someone, you don't really have to pay such close attention to them any more.
- ❑ **2B.** Recognize that closeness is built by attending to and learning more and more about people you care about.

- ❑ **3A.** "My feelings are really hurt by what you did, and the thought went through my mind that you hate me. I know that you don't really, but did you feel that way at the time?"
- ❑ **3B.** "I know you hate me. There is no other reason for what you did to me. Don't tell me differently, either."

- ❑ **4A.** In social situations, throw yourself into interactions.
- ❑ **4B.** Stay reserved and watch social interactions so you don't make mistakes.

- ❑ **5A.** Find people with your values.
- ❑ **5B.** Do little immoral things so as not to be a drag on friendships.

- ❑ **6A.** Be open to people's changing their minds about things, as well as their beliefs or feelings.
- ❑ **6B.** Assume that when people change, they are not trustworthy.

- ❑ **7A.** Evaluate other people's behaviors and thoughts, and tell them that they are wrong or that they should be different when you feel sure you are right.
- ❑ **7B.** If you do not approve of or agree with what another person is doing or thinking, try to understand how it would make sense if you knew the causes.

- ❑ **8A.** "You should stop doing that."
- ❑ **8B.** "I wish you would stop doing that."

- ❑ **9A.** "You are lazy and have given up."
- ❑ **9B.** "I worry that you have given up."

- ❑ **10A.** "I don't think that is correct."
- ❑ **10B.** "How could you possibly think that?"

- ❑ **11A.** Stay in control so that relationships turn out the way you want.
- ❑ **11B.** Go with the flow much of the time when in social interactions with groups of friends.

- ❑ **12A.** Hold back in a conversation until you are sure you like the person.
- ❑ **12B.** Throw yourself into a conversation until you are sure you don't like it.

Ending Relationships

A destructive relationship has the quality of destroying or completely spoiling either the quality of the relationship or aspects of yourself—such as your physical body and safety, your self-esteem or sense of integrity, your happiness or peace of mind, or your caring for the other person.

An interfering relationship is one that blocks or makes difficult your pursuing goals that are important to you; your ability to enjoy life and do things you like doing; your relationships with other persons; or the welfare of others that you love.

> **Decide to end relationships in WISE MIND,
> NEVER in emotion mind.**

> **If the relationship is IMPORTANT and NOT destructive,
> and there is reason to hope it can be improved, try
> PROBLEM SOLVING to repair a difficult relationship.**

> **COPE AHEAD to troubleshoot
> and practice ending the relationship ahead of time.**

> **Be direct: Use the DEAR MAN GIVE FAST interpersonal
> effectiveness skills.**

> **Practice OPPOSITE ACTION FOR LOVE when you find
> you love the wrong person.**

> **PRACTICE SAFETY FIRST!
> Before leaving a highly abusive or life-threatening
> relationship, call a local domestic violence hotline or the
> toll-free National Domestic Violence Hotline (1-800-799-7233)
> for help with safety planning and a referral to a qualified
> professional. See also the International Directory of Domestic
> Violence Agencies (*www.hotpeachpages.net*).**

Identifying How to End Relationships

For each A and B pair, check the more effective response.

☐ **1A.** If a relationship is threatening your integrity or physical well-being, it is probably your fault, and you should see a therapist.

☐ **1B.** A relationship threatening your integrity or physical well-being is destructive, and you should consider getting out of it.

In the middle of an argument, you are so mad at the other person you don't want to have anything to do with this person any more.

☐ **5A.** You should end the relationship right then! You may forget all about how enraging the person is if you wait.

☐ **5B.** You should get out of emotion mind and into Wise Mind, and evaluate whether to stay or leave the relationship.

☐ **2A.** Relationships should be easy. If it's hard to have a relationship with someone, it's probably not worth it, and you should end it.

☐ **2B.** Most relationships need problem solving to work.

☐ **6A.** If ending a destructive relationship will be difficult, it's most effective to stay together.

☐ **6B.** If ending a destructive relationship will be difficult, it's most effective to cope ahead of time.

☐ **3A.** If you are in love with someone who does not love you back, practice DEAR MAN skills to get the person to love you.

☐ **3B.** If you are in love with someone who does not love you back, practice opposite action to love.

☐ **7A.** In an abusive relationship, if the person hits you, you should use your interpersonal skills to tell the person you are leaving the relationship.

☐ **7B.** In an abusive relationship, you should seek professional assistance to leave the relationship.

☐ **4A.** To decide whether to end a relationship, do PROS and CONS.

☐ **4B.** To decide whether to end a relationship, use GIVE skills.

☐ **8A.** If you feel consistently invalidated in a relationship, it is probably your fault.

☐ **8B.** If you are consistently invalidated, the relationship is likely destructive.

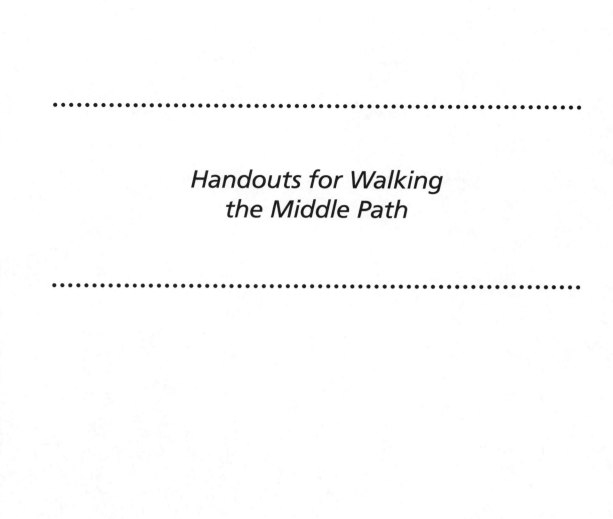

*Handouts for Walking
the Middle Path*

Overview:
Walking the Middle Path

Balancing Acceptance and Change

DIALECTICS

Balancing opposites while entering the paradox of "yes"
and "no," "true" and "not true," at the very same time.

VALIDATION

Including the valid and understanable in ourselves and others.

RECOVERING FROM INVALIDATION

From a nondefensive position, find the valid, acknowledge
the invalid, and radically accept yourself.

STRATEGIES FOR CHANGING BEHAVIOR

Use behavioral principles to increase desired behaviors and
decrease undesired behaviors.

Dialectics

DIALECTICS REMINDS US THAT

1. The universe is filled with opposing sides/opposing forces.

There is always more than one way to see a situation, and more than one way to solve a problem.

Two things that seem like opposites can both be true.

2. Everything and every person is connected in some way.

The waves and the ocean are one.

The slightest move of the butterfly affects the furthest star.

3. Change is the only constant.

Meaning and truth evolve over time.

Each moment is new; reality itself changes with each moment.

4. Change is transactional.

What we do influences our environment and other people in it.

The environment and other people influence us.

How to Think and Act Dialectically

☐ 1. **There is always more than one side to anything that exists. Look for both sides.**

  ☐ **Ask Wise Mind: What am I missing?** Where is the kernel of truth in the other side?

  ☐ **Let go of extremes:** Change "either-or" to "both-and," "always" or "never" to "sometimes."

  ☐ **Balance opposites:** Validate both sides when you disagree, accept reality, and work to change.

  ☐ **Make lemonade out of lemons.**

  ☐ **Embrace confusion:** Enter the paradox of yes and no, or true and not true.

  ☐ **Play devil's advocate:** Argue each side of your own position with equal passion.

  ☐ **Use metaphors and storytelling** to unstick and free the mind.

  ☐ **Other ways to see all sides of a situation:** _____

☐ 2. **Be aware that you are connected.**

  ☐ **Treat others as you want them to treat you.**

  ☐ **Look for similarities among people instead of differences.**

  ☐ **Notice the physical connections** among all things.

  ☐ **Other ways to stay aware of connections:** _____

☐ 3. **Embrace change.**

  ☐ **Throw yourself into change:** Allow it. Embrace it.

  ☐ **Practice radical acceptance of change** when rules, circumstances, people, and relationships change in ways you don't like.

  ☐ **Practice getting used to change:** Make small changes to practice this (e.g., purposely change where you sit, who you talk with, what route you take when going to a familiar place).

  ☐ **Other ways to embrace change:** _____

☐ 4. **Change is transactional: Remember that you affect your environment and your environment affects you.**

  ☐ **Pay attention to your effect on others** and how they affect you.

  ☐ **Practice letting go of blame** by looking for how your own and others' behaviors are caused by many interactions over time.

  ☐ **Remind yourself that all things, including all behaviors, are caused.**

  ☐ **Other ways to see transactions:** _____

Examples of Opposite Sides That Can Both Be True

❑ 1. You can want to change and be doing the best you can, AND still need to do better, try harder, and be more motivated to change.

❑ 2. You are tough AND you are gentle.

❑ 3. You can be independent AND also want help. (You can allow somebody else to be independent AND also give them help.)

❑ 4. You can want to be alone AND also want to be connected to others.

❑ 5. You can share some things with others AND also keep some things private.

❑ 6. You can be by yourself AND still be connected to others.

❑ 7. You can be with others AND be lonely.

❑ 8. You can be a misfit in one group AND fit in perfectly in another group. (A tulip in a rose garden can also be a tulip in a tulip garden.)

❑ 9. You can accept yourself the way you are AND still want to change. (You can accept others as they are AND still want them to change.)

❑ 10. At times you need to both control AND tolerate your emotions.

❑ 11. You may have a valid reason for believing what you believe, AND you may still be wrong or incorrect.

❑ 12. Someone may have valid reasons for wanting something from you, AND you may have valid reasons for saying no.

❑ 13. The day can be sunny, AND it can rain.

❑ 14. You can be mad at somebody AND also love and respect the person.

❑ 15. (You can be mad at yourself AND also love and respect yourself.)

❑ 16. You can have a disagreement with somebody AND also be friends.

❑ 17. You can disagree with the rules AND also follow the rules.

❑ 18. You can understand why somebody is feeling or behaving in a certain way, AND also disagree with his or her behavior and ask that it be changed.

❑ 19. Others: _____

Important Opposites to Balance

❑ 1. Accepting reality AND working to change it.

❑ 2. Validating yourself and others AND acknowledging errors.

❑ 3. Working AND resting.

❑ 4. Doing things you need to do AND doing things you want to do.

❑ 5. Working on improving yourself AND accepting yourself exactly as you are.

❑ 6. Problem solving AND problem acceptance.

❑ 7. Emotion regulation AND emotion acceptance.

❑ 8. Mastering something on your own AND asking for help.

❑ 9. Independence AND dependence.

❑ 10. Openness AND privacy.

❑ 11. Trust AND suspicion.

❑ 12. Watching and observing AND participating.

❑ 13. Taking from others AND giving to others.

❑ 14. Focusing on yourself AND focusing on others.

❑ 15. Others: _____

_____

❑ 16. Others: _____

_____

❑ 17. Others: _____

_____

Identifying Dialectics

For each group, check the most dialectical response.

☐ **1A.** Pay attention to your effect on others.

☐ **1B.** Assume that others' reactions to you are unrelated to your treatment of them.

☐ **5A.** Examine a difficult relationship by looking at how the interactions over time between you and the other person may be problematic.

☐ **5B.** Assume that difficulties in a relationship are caused completely by you or by the other person.

Saying:

☐ **2A.** "I know I am right about this."

☐ **2B.** "I can see your point of view, even though I do not agree with it."

☐ **2C.** "The way you are thinking doesn't make any sense."

Saying:

☐ **6A.** "It is hopeless. I cannot do it."

☐ **6B.** "This is a breeze. I've got no problems."

☐ **6C.** "This is really hard for me, and I am going to keep trying."

Saying:

☐ **3A.** "Everyone always treats me unfairly."

☐ **3B.** "I believe the coach should reconsider his decision to cut me from the team."

☐ **3C.** "Coaches know best who to keep on teams and who to cut."

☐ **7A.** When you disagree with someone, be sure and be very clear about your point of view.

☐ **7B.** When you disagree with someone, try and see their point of view.

☐ **4A.** Judge friends as disloyal and uncaring if they start changing in ways you don't like.

☐ **4B.** Accept that interests change.

☐ **8A.** Demand that relationships be stable without changing.

☐ **8B.** Embrace change and see it as inevitable.

Note. Adapted in part from Miller, A. L., Rathus, J. H., & Linehan, M. M. (2007). *Dialectical behavior therapy with suicidal adolescents.* New York: Guilford Press. Copyright 2007 by The Guilford Press. Adapted by permission.

Validation

VALIDATION MEANS:

- Finding the kernel of truth in another person's perspective or situation; verifying the facts of a situation.
- Acknowledging that a person's emotions, thoughts, and behaviors have causes and are therefore understandable.
- *Not* necessarily agreeing with the other person.
- *Not* validating what is actually invalid.

WHY VALIDATE?

- It improves our relationships by showing we are listening and understand.
- It improves interpersonal effectiveness by reducing:
    1. Pressure to prove who is right
    2. Negative reactivity
    3. Anger
- It makes problem solving, closeness, and support possible.
- Invalidation hurts.

IMPORTANT THINGS TO VALIDATE

- The valid (and *only* the valid).
- The facts of a situation.
- A person's experiences, feelings/emotions, beliefs, opinions, or thoughts about something.
- Suffering and difficulties.

REMEMBER:

- Every invalid response makes sense in some way.
- Validation is not necessarily agreeing.
- Validation doesn't mean you like it.
- Only validate the valid!

Note. Adapted from Linehan, M. M. (1997). Validation and psychotherapy. In A. Bohart & L. Greenberg (Eds.), *Empathy reconsidered: New directions in psychotherapy* (pp. 353–392). Washington, DC: American Psychological Association. Copyright 1997 by the American Psychological Association. Adapted by permission.

A "How To" Guide to Validation

1. ❑ **Pay Attention:**
   Look interested, listen, and observe. No multitasking. Make eye contact. Stay focused. Nod occasionally. Respond with your face (e.g., smile at happy statements; look concerned when hearing something painful).

2. ❑ **Reflect Back:**
   Say back what you heard or observed to be sure you actually understand what the person is saying. *No* judgmental language or voice tone!

   Try to really "get" what the person feels or thinks. Have an open mind. (No disagreeing, criticizing, or trying to change the person's mind or goals.) Use a voice tone that allows the other person to correct you . . . and *check the facts!*

   Example: *"So you are mad at me because you think I lied just to get back at you. Did I get it right?"*

3. ❑ **"Read Minds":**
   Be sensitive to what is *not* being said by the other person. Pay attention to facial expressions, body language, what is happening, and what you know about the person already. Show that you understand in words or by your actions. *Be open to correction.*

   Example: *When you are asking a friend for a ride at the end of a long day and the person slumps down, say, "You look really tired. Let me look for someone else."*

4. ❑ **Understand:**
   Look for how the other person feels, is thinking, or if he or she is making sense, given the person's history, state of mind or body, or current events (i.e. the causes)—even if you don't approve of the person's behavior, or if his or her belief is incorrect. Say *"It makes sense that you . . . because . . . "*

   Example: *If you sent a party invitation to the wrong address, say, "I can see why you thought I might be excluding you on purpose."*

5. ❑ **Acknowledge the valid:**
   Show that you see that the person's thoughts, feelings, or actions are valid, given current reality and facts. Act as if the person's behavior is valid.

   Example: *If you are criticized for not taking out the garbage on your day, admit that it is your day and take it out. If people present a problem, help them solve it (unless they just want to be heard). If people are hungry, give them food. Acknowledge the effort a person is making.*

6. ❑ **Show Equality:**
   Be yourself! Don't "one-up" or "one-down" the other person. Treat the other as an equal, not as fragile or incompetent.

   Example: *Be willing to admit mistakes. If someone introduces him- or herself by first name, introduce yourself by your first name. Ask other people for their opinions. Give up being defensive. Be careful in giving advice or telling someone what to do if you are not asked or required to do so. Even then, remember you could be wrong.*

Note. Adapted from Linehan, M. M. (1997). Validation and psychotherapy. In A. Bohart & L. Greenberg (Eds.), *Empathy reconsidered: New directions in psychotherapy* (pp. 353–392). Washington, DC: American Psychological Association. Copyright 1997 by the American Psychological Association. Adapted by permission.

Identifying Validation

For each A and B pair, check the more effective response.

❑ **1A.** Think about your day when the other person is talking about his or her day.

❑ **1B.** Throw yourself into listening about the other person's day.

❑ **5A.** Remember that people's thoughts, feelings, and behaviors don't always match. Check the facts.

❑ **5B.** Assume that you can tell exactly what people are feeling and thinking.

❑ **2A.** If you are uncertain of people's thoughts and feelings, ask them what they are thinking or feeling, or try to imagine yourself in their situation.

❑ **2B.** Assume that if people want you to know what they are thinking or feeling, they will tell you.

❑ **6A.** Evaluate other people's behaviors and thoughts, and tell them that they are wrong or that they should be different when you feel sure you are right.

❑ **6B.** If you do not agree with what another person is doing or thinking, try to understand how it could make sense if you understood the causes.

❑ **3A.** Observe the small clues that indicate what is going on in social situations.

❑ **3B.** Observe only what people say, and ignore nonverbal signals.

❑ **7A.** Assume that if you tell a person his or her request of you makes sense, that's all you have to do to validate the person.

❑ **7B.** When a person asks you for something, giving the person what has been asked for is validation.

❑ **4A.** Jump to conclusions about what people mean.

❑ **4B.** Realize that the same behavior can mean many things.

❑ **8A.** Assume that other people's reactions to you have nothing to do with yours to them.

❑ **8B.** Treat each person with respect and as an equal.

Recovering from Invalidation

NOTICE THAT INVALIDATION
CAN BE HELPFUL AND PAINFUL AT THE SAME TIME

Remember:
Invalidation Is Helpful When

1. It corrects important mistakes (your facts are wrong).

2. It stimulates intellectual and personal growth by listening to other views.

3. Other: _____

Invalidation Is Painful When

1. You are being ignored.

2. You are not being repeatedly misunderstood.

3. You are being misread.

4. You are being misinterpreted.

5. Important facts in your life are ignored or denied.

6. You are receiving unequal treatment.

7. You are being disbelieved when being truthful.

8. Your private experiences are trivialized or denied.

9. Other: _____

---

*(**continued on next page**)*

Be Nondefensive and Check the Facts

❑ Check ALL the facts to see if your responses are valid or invalid. Check them out with someone you can trust to validate the valid.

❑ Acknowledge when your responses don't make sense and are not valid.

❑ Work to change invalid thinking, comments, or actions. (Also, stop blaming. It rarely helps a situation.)

❑ Drop judgmental self-statements. (Practice opposite action.)

❑ Remind yourself that all behavior is caused and that you are doing your best.

❑ Be compassionate toward yourself. Practice self-soothing.

❑ Admit that it hurts to be invalidated by others, even if they are right.

❑ Acknowledge when your reactions make sense and are valid in a situation.

❑ Remember that being invalidated, even when your response is actually valid, is rarely a complete catastrophe.

❑ Describe your experiences and actions in a supportive environment.

❑ Grieve traumatic invalidation and the harm it created.

❑ Practice radical acceptance of the invalidating person.

Validate Yourself Exactly the Way You Would Validate Someone Else

Identifying Self-Validation

For each A and B pair, check the more effective response when someone else invalidates you.

❑ **1A.** Describe your own experience, point of view, emotion, or action in a matter-of-fact way.

❑ **1B.** Say, "How stupid of me," or put yourself down for your response.

❑ **2A.** Blast the other person and argue your point of view, even if you might be wrong.

❑ **2B.** When someone disagrees with what you think or do, be open to being wrong and being OK with that. Check the facts.

❑ **3A.** When you are checking the facts (if only in your mind), stand up for yourself if you are correct or if your response is reasonable.

❑ **3B.** Assume that your experience of the facts is wrong. Give up and give in. Judge yourself and the person who invalidated you.

❑ **4A.** Jump to anger and call yourself a wimp if you start feeling sad or alone.

❑ **4B.** Accept that it hurts to be invalidated, and feel the pain.

❑ **5A.** When you make a mistake, remind yourself that you are human, and humans make mistakes.

❑ **5B.** Blame and punish yourself for being wrong; avoid people who know you were wrong.

❑ **6A.** See yourself as "screwed up" or "damaged goods," and give in to shame and misery.

❑ **6B.** Respond and talk to yourself with understanding and compassion. Remind yourself that all responses are caused and make sense if you explore the reasons long enough.

Strategies for Increasing the Probability
of Behaviors You Want

Describe behaviors for yourself or others that you would like to start or increase:

_____

Reinforcer = A consequence that increases frequency of a behavior.

Positive reinforcement = positive consequences (i.e., reward).

Behavior is increased by consequences a person wants, likes, or will work to get.

Examples: _____

Negative reinforcement = removal of negative events (i.e., relief).

Behavior is increased by consequences that stop or reduce something negative.

Examples: _____

Shaping = Reinforcing small steps toward the behavior you want.

- Reinforce small steps that lead toward the goal.
- As new behavior stabilizes, require a little bit more before reinforcing.
- Continue until you reach the goal behavior.

Examples of steps to a goal behavior: _____

_____

Timing counts.

- Reinforce behavior immediately after it occurs.
- When shaping new behavior, at first reinforce every instance of the behavior.
- Once behavior is established, gradually start to reinforce only some of the time.

CAUTION: When you vary reinforcement, behavior becomes *very* hard to stop.

Strategies for Decreasing or Stopping Unwanted Behaviors

Extinction = Stopping an ongoing reinforcement of behavior.

Extinction leads first to a burst of behavior, and then to a decrease in behavior.

Examples: _____

Satiation = Providing relief or what is wanted *before* the behavior occurs.

Satiation reduces motivation for behavior and thus decreases its frequency.

Examples: _____

Punishment = An aversive consequence that decreases a behavior.

Behavior is decreased by consequences the person dislikes or will work to avoid.

Examples: _____

Behavior is decreased by consequences that stop or reduce something positive.

Examples: _____

Behavior is decreased when something the person wants is withheld until harmful effects of problem behaviors are corrected and overcorrected.

Examples: _____

- Be sure that punishment is specific, is time-limited, and fits the "crime."
- Avoid a punitive tone; let the consequence do the work.
- If a natural punishment occurs, don't undo it. Don't add arbitrary punishment.

Be sure to reinforce alternative behavior to replace behavior you want stopped.

- Extinction and punishment weaken or suppress behavior, but do not eliminate it.
- Extinction and punishment do not teach new behavior.
- To keep a behavior from resurfacing, reinforce an alternative behavior.
- Punishment works only when the punisher is (or is likely to be) present.
- Punishment leads to avoidance of the person punishing.

Tips for Using Behavior Change Strategies Effectively

Summary so far:

Goal		Consequence
Increase behavior	(Reinforce)	• Add positive consequence • Remove aversive consequence
Weaken behavior	(Extinguish)	• Remove reinforcer • Provide relief *before* unwanted behavior
Suppress behavior	(Punish)	• Add aversive consequence • Remove positive consequence

---

Not all consequences are created equal.

"One person's poison can be another person's passion."

Context counts. A reinforcer in one situation can be punishment in another.

Quantity counts. If a reinforcer is too little or too much, it will not work.

Natural consequences work best. Let them do the work when possible.

Ask what consequence the person would work to get (reinforcer) or work to avoid (punisher).

Observe changes in behavior when a consequence is applied.

Behavior learned in one situation may not happen in another situation.

Identifying Effective Behavior Change Strategies

For each A and B pair, check the more effective response.

❑ **1A.** When you are trying to increase a behavior, it is most effective to wait for the full desired behavior before reinforcing, so the person does not think that halfway is good enough.

❑ **1B.** When you are trying to increase a behavior, it is most effective to reinforce small improvement in the right direction, or else the person may not continue to improve.

❑ **2A.** The most effective punishment is intense anger and swift verbal criticism.

❑ **2B.** The most effective punishment is to find one that fits the severity of the problem behavior.

❑ **3A.** It is most effective to reinforce behavior immediately after it occurs.

❑ **3B.** It is most effective to reward behavior after a delay so that the person does not expect that you will always provide a reward.

❑ **4A.** It is common that people reward others' problematic behaviors without even realizing it.

❑ **4B.** People do not reward others' problematic behaviors, because that would be stupid.

❑ **5A.** If a person's problem behaviors work to get things he or she wants, it is most effective to punish those behaviors to make them stop.

❑ **5B.** If a person's problem behaviors work to get things he or she wants, it is most effective to stop reinforcing those behaviors and instead give rewards when the person uses more skillful strategies to get what he or she wants or needs.

❑ **6A.** When you are punishing, figure that a nonspecific punishment will be a lot more effective, since it can't be avoided.

❑ **6B.** Use a specific and time-limited negative consequence to decrease behavior.

❑ **7A.** If a person's mean behavior makes you feel hurt, it is most effective to punish the behavior by taking away gifts that you previously gave the person.

❑ **7B.** If a person's mean behavior makes you feel hurt, it is most effective to punish the behavior by not doing favors for the person until his or her behavior improves.

❑ **8A.** After a punished behavior stops, it is most effective to reward an alternative behavior that you want.

❑ **8B.** After a punished behavior stops, it is most effective to continue the punishment, so that you send a very clear message that the problematic behavior is unacceptable.

Interpersonal Effectiveness Worksheets

Worksheets for Goals and Factors That Interfere

Pros and Cons of Using Interpersonal Effectiveness Skills

Due Date: _____   Name: _____ Week Starting: _____

Use this sheet to figure out the advantages and disadvantages to you of using interpersonal effectiveness skills (i.e., acting skillfully) to get what you want. The idea here is to figure out what is the most effective way for you to get what you want. Remember, this is about your goals, not someone else's goals.

Describe the interpersonal situation:

_____

_____

Describe your goal in this situation:

_____

_____

Make a list of the pros and cons of acting skillfully by using interpersonal effectiveness skills.

Make another list of the pros and cons for using power tactics to get what you want.

Make a third list of pros and cons for giving in or acting passively in the situation.

Check the facts to be sure that you are correct in your assessment of advantages and disadvantages.

Write on the back of this sheet if you need more room.

	Using Skills	Demanding, Attacking, Stonewalling	Giving In, Acting Passively
PROS	_____ _____ _____	_____ _____ _____	_____ _____ _____
CONS	_____ _____ _____	_____ _____ _____	_____ _____ _____

What did you decide to do in this situation? _____

_____

Is this the best decision (in Wise Mind)? _____

_____

Challenging Myths in the Way of Obtaining Objectives

Challenging Myths in the Way of Objectives Effectiveness

Due Date: _____ Name: _____ Week Starting: _____

For each myth, write down a challenge that makes sense to you.

1. I don't deserve to get what I want or need.

   Challenge: _____

2. If I make a request, this will show that I'm a very weak person.

   Challenge: _____

3. I have to know whether a person is going to say yes before I make a request.

   Challenge: _____

4. If I ask for something or say no, I can't stand it if someone gets upset with me.

   Challenge: _____

5. If they say no, it will kill me.

   Challenge: _____

6. Making requests is a really pushy (bad, self-centered, selfish, etc.) thing to do.

   Challenge: _____

7. Saying no to a request is always a selfish thing to do.

   Challenge: _____

8. I should be willing to sacrifice my own needs for others.

   Challenge: _____

9. I must be really inadequate if I can't fix this myself.

   Challenge: _____

10. Obviously, the problem is just in my head. If I would just think differently, I wouldn't have to bother everybody else.

    Challenge: _____

11. If I don't have what I want or need, it doesn't make any difference; I don't care, really.

    Challenge: _____

12. Skillfulness is a sign of weakness.

    Challenge: _____

    Other myth: _____

    Challenge: _____

    Other myth: _____

    Challenge: _____

(*continued on next page*)

Challenging Myths in the Way of Relationship and Self-Respect Effectiveness

For each myth, write down a challenge that makes sense to you.

13. I shouldn't have to ask (say no); they should know what I want (and do it).

    Challenge: _____

14. They should have known that their behavior would hurt my feelings; I shouldn't have to tell them.

    Challenge: _____

15. I shouldn't have to negotiate or work at getting what I want.

    Challenge: _____

16. Other people should be willing to do more for my needs.

    Challenge: _____

17. Other people should like, approve of, and support me.

    Challenge: _____

18. They don't deserve my being skillful or treating them well.

    Challenge: _____

19. Getting what I want when I want it is most important.

    Challenge: _____

20. I shouldn't be fair, kind, courteous, or respectful if others are not so toward me.

    Challenge: _____

21. Revenge will feel so good; it will be worth any negative consequences.

    Challenge: _____

22. Only wimps have values.

    Challenge: _____

23. Everybody lies.

    Challenge: _____

24. Getting what I want or need is more important than how I get it; the ends really do justify the means.

    Challenge: _____

    Other myth: _____

    Challenge: _____

    Other myth: _____

    Challenge: _____

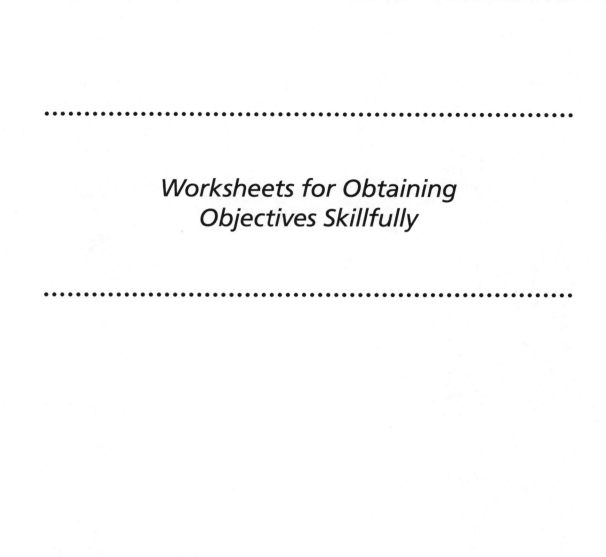

Worksheets for Obtaining Objectives Skillfully

Clarifying Priorities in Interpersonal Situations

Due Date: _____   Name: _____ Week Starting: _____

Use this sheet to figure out your goals and priorities in any situation that creates a problem for you. Examples include situations where (1) your rights or wishes are not being respected; (2) you want someone to do or change something or give you something; (3) you want or need to say no or resist pressure to do something; (4) you want to get your position or point of view taken seriously; (5) there is conflict with another person; or (6) you want to improve your relationship with someone.

Observe and describe in writing as close in time to the situation as possible. Write on the back of this sheet if you need more room.

Prompting event for my problem: Who did what to whom? What led up to what?
What is it about this situation that is a problem for me?
Remember to **check the facts!**

My wants and desires in this situation:

Objectives: What **specific results** do I want? What do I want this person to do, stop or accept?

Relationship: How do I want the other person to feel and think about me **because of how I handle the interaction** (whether or not I get what I want from the other person)?

Self-Respect: How do I want to feel or think about myself **because of how I handle the interaction** (whether or not I get what I want from the other person)?

My priorities in this situation: Rate priorities 1 (most important), 2 (second most important), or 3 (least important).

____Objectives   ____Relationship   ____Self-respect

Imbalances and conflicts in priorities that make it hard to be effective in this situation:

Writing Out Interpersonal Effectiveness Scripts

Due Date: _____   Name: _____ Week Starting: _____

Fill out this sheet before you practice your DEAR MAN, GIVE FAST interpersonal skills. Practice saying your "lines" out loud, and also in your mind. Use the "cope ahead" skills (Emotion Regulation Handout 19). Write on the back of this sheet if you need more room.

PROMPTING EVENT for my problem: Who did what to whom? What led up to what?

OBJECTIVES IN SITUATION (What results I want):

RELATIONSHIP ISSUE (How I want the other person to feel about me):

SELF-RESPECT ISSUE (How I want to feel about myself):

SCRIPT IDEAS for DEAR MAN, GIVE FAST

1. **Describe** situation.

2. **Express** feelings/opinions.

3. **Assert** request (or say no) directly (circle the part you will use later in "broken record" to stay **M**indful if you need it).

4. **Reinforcing** comments to make.

5. **Mindful and Appearing** confident comments to make (if needed).

6 **Negotiating** comments to make, plus turn-the-table comments (if needed).

7. **Validating** comments.

8. **Easy manner** comments.

Write on the back side all the things you want to *avoid* doing and saying.

Tracking Interpersonal Effectiveness Skills Use

Due Date: _____   Name: _____   Week Starting: _____

Fill out this sheet whenever you practice your interpersonal skills and whenever you have an opportunity to practice, even if you don't (or almost don't) do anything to practice. Write on the back of this sheet if you need more room.

PROMPTING EVENT for my problem: Who did what to whom? What led up to what?

OBJECTIVES IN SITUATION (What results I want):

RELATIONSHIP ISSUE (How I want the other person to feel about me):

SELF-RESPECT ISSUE (How I want to feel about myself):

My PRIORITIES in this situation: Rate priorities 1 (most important), 2 (second most important), or 3 (least important).

_____OBJECTIVES   _____RELATIONSHIP   _____SELF-RESPECT

Imbalances and CONFLICTS IN PRIORITIES that made it hard to be effective in this situation:

What I SAID OR DID in the situation: (Describe and check below.)

DEAR MAN (Getting what I want):
_____ Described situation?_____
_____ Expressed feelings/opinions?_____
_____ Asserted?_____
_____ Reinforced?_____

_____ Mindful?_____
_____ Broken record?_____
_____ Ignored attacks?_____
_____ Appeared confident?_____
_____ Negotiated?_____

GIVE (Keeping the relationship):
_____ Gentle?_____
_____ No threats?_____
_____ No attacks?_____
_____ No judgments?_____

_____ Interested?_____
_____ Validated?_____
_____ Easy manner?_____

FAST (Keeping my respect for myself):
_____ Fair?_____
_____ (No) Apologies?_____

_____ Stuck to values?_____
_____ Truthful?_____

How effective was the interaction? _____
_____

INTERPERSONAL EFFECTIVENESS WORKSHEET 6 (I. E. Handout 8) (p. 1 of 2)

The Dime Game: Figuring Out How Strongly to Ask or Say No

Due Date: _____   Name: _____   Week Starting: _____

To figure out how strongly to ask for something or how strongly to say no, read the instructions below. Circle the dimes you put in the bank, and then add them up. Then go back over the list and see if some items are much more important than others. Check Wise Mind before acting, if some items are much more important than others.

Decide how strongly to ask for something.

Put a dime in the bank for each of the questions that get a yes answer. The more money you have, the stronger you ask. If you have a dollar, then ask very strongly. If you don't have any money in the bank, then don't ask; don't even hint.

Decide how strongly to say no.

Put a dime in the bank for each of the questions that get a no answer. The more money you have, the stronger you say no. If you have a dollar, then say no very strongly. If you don't have any money in the bank, then do it without even hint.

Ask		Category		Say No
10¢	Is this person able to give or do what I want?	**Capability**	Can I give the person what is wanted?	10¢
10¢	Is getting my objective more important than my relationship with this person?	**Priorities**	Is my relationship more important than saying no?	10¢
10¢	Will asking help me feel competent and self-respecting?	**Self-respect**	Will saying no make me feel bad about myself?	10¢
10¢	Is the person required by law or moral code to do or give me what I want?	**Rights**	Am I required by law or moral code to give or do what is wanted, or does saying no violate this person's rights?	10¢
10¢	Am I responsible for telling the person what to do?	**Authority**	Is the other person responsible for telling me what to do?	10¢
10¢	Is what I want appropriate for this relationship? (Is it right to ask for what I want?)	**Relationship**	Is what the person is requesting of me appropriate to my relationship with this person?	10¢
10¢	Is asking important to a long-term goal?	**Goals**	In the long term, will I regret saying no?	10¢
10¢	Do I give as much as I get with this person?	**Give and take**	Do I owe this person a favor? (Does the person do a lot for me?)	10¢
10¢	Do I know what I want and have the facts I need to support my request?	**Homework**	Do I know what I am saying no to? (Is the other person clear about what is being asked for?)	10¢
10¢	Is this a good time to ask? (Is the person in the right mood?)	**Timing**	Should I wait a while before saying no?	10¢
$	**Total value of asking** (Adjusted ± ___ for Wise Mind)	**Total value of saying no** (Adjusted ± ___ for Wise Mind)		$

(continued on next page)

ASKING		SAYING NO
Don't ask; don't hint.	0–10¢	Do it without being asked.
Hint indirectly; take no.	20¢	Don't complain; do it cheerfully.
Hint openly; take no.	30¢	Do it, even if you're not cheerful about it.
Ask tentatively; take no.	40¢	Do it, but show that you'd rather not.
Ask gracefully, but take no.	50¢	Say you'd rather not, but do it gracefully.
Ask confidently; take no.	60¢	Say no firmly, but reconsider.
Ask confidently; resist no.	70¢	Say no confidently; resist saying yes.
Ask firmly; resist no.	80¢	Say no firmly; resist saying yes.
Ask firmly; insist; negotiate; keep trying.	90¢	Say no firmly; resist; negotiate.
Don't take no for an answer.	$1.00	Don't do it.

Troubleshooting Interpersonal Effectiveness Skills

Due Date: _____ Name: _____ Week Starting: _____

Fill out this sheet whenever you practice your interpersonal skills and whenever you have an opportunity to practice, even if you don't (or almost don't) do anything to practice. Write on the back of this sheet if you need more room.

Do I have the skills I need? Check out the instructions.

1 Review what has already been tried.
- Do I know how to be skillful in getting what I want?
- Do I know how to say what I want to say?
- Did I follow the skill instructions to the letter?

❑ **Not sure:**
  ❑ Wrote out what I wanted to say first.
  ❑ Reread the instructions.
  ❑ Got coaching from someone I trust.
  ❑ Practiced with a friend or in front of a mirror.
    Did it work the next time? ❑ Yes (Fabulous) ❑ No (Continue) ❑ Didn't try again
❑ **Yes:**

Do I know what I really want in this interaction?

2 Ask:
- Am I undecided about what I really want in this interaction?
- Am I ambivalent about my priorities?
- Am I having trouble balancing:
  - Asking for too much versus not asking for anything?
  - Saying no to everything versus giving in to everything?
- Is fear or shame getting in the way of knowing what I really want?

❑ **Not sure:**
  ❑ Did pros and cons to compare different objectives.
  ❑ Used emotion regulation skills to reduce fear and shame.
    Did this help? ❑ Yes (Fabulous) ❑ No (Continue) ❑ Didn't try again
❑ **Yes:**

Are my short-term goals getting in the way of my long-term goals?

3 Ask:
- Is "now, now, now" winning out over getting what I really want?
- Is emotion mind controlling what I say and do instead of Wise Mind?

❑ **Yes:**
  ❑ Did a pros and cons comparing short-term to long-term goals.
  ❑ Waited until another time when I'm not in emotion mind.
    Did this help? ❑ Yes (Fabulous) ❑ No (Continue) ❑ Didn't try again
❑ **No:**

(*continued on next page*)

Are my emotions getting in the way of using my skills?

4 Ask:
- Do I get too upset to use my skills?
- Are my emotions so high that I am over my skills breakdown point?

❏ **Yes:**
  ❏ Tried *TIP* skills.
  ❏ Used self-soothing crisis survival skills before the interaction to get myself calm.
  ❏ Did mindfulness of current emotions (Emotion Regulation Handout 22).
  ❏ Refocused attention completely on the present objective.
    Did this help? ❏ Yes (Fabulous) ❏ No (Continue) ❏ Didn't try again
❏ **No:**

Are worries, assumptions, and myths getting in my way?

5 Ask:
- Are thoughts about bad consequences blocking my action?
  "They won't like me," "She will think I am stupid."
- Are thoughts about whether I deserve to get what I want in my way?
  "I am such a bad person I don't deserve this."
- Am I calling myself names that stop me from doing anything?
  "I won't do it right," "I'll probably fall apart," "I'm so stupid."
- Am I believing myths about interpersonal effectiveness?
  "If I make a request, this will show that I am a very weak person," "Only wimps have values."

❏ **Yes:**
  ❏ Challenged myths.
  ❏ Checked the facts.
  ❏ Did opposite action all the way.
    Did this help? ❏ Yes (Fabulous) ❏ No (Continue) ❏ Didn't try again
❏ **No:**

Is the environment more powerful than my skills?

6 Ask:
- Are the people who have what I want or need more powerful than I am?
- Are the people commanding me powerful and in control?
- Will others be threatened if I get what I want?
- Do others have reasons for not liking me if I get what I want?

❏ **Yes:**
  ❏ Tried problem solving.
  ❏ Found a powerful ally.
  ❏ Practiced radical acceptance.
    Did this help? ❏ Yes (Fabulous) ❏ No (Continue) ❏ Didn't try again
❏ **No:**

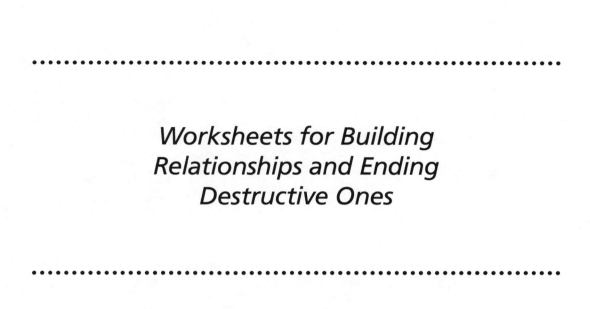

*Worksheets for Building
Relationships and Ending
Destructive Ones*

Finding and Getting People to Like You

Due Date: _____ Name: _____ Week Starting: _____

Fill out this sheet whenever you practice finding friends and whenever you have an opportunity to practice, even if you don't (or almost don't) do anything to practice. Write on the back of this sheet if you need more room.

List two ways you could (or do) make casual but regular contact with people.

1. _____

2. _____

List two ways you could find (or have found) people whose attitudes are similar to yours.

1. _____

2. _____

List two ways you could get in conversations (or have been in them) where you could ask a question, give an answer, give a compliment, or express liking to others.

1. _____

2. _____

List times you have been near a group conversation you could practice joining (or how you could find one).

1. _____

2. _____

Check the facts and be sure you have listed all of your opportunities to find potential friends. Add more ideas if necessary or ask your current friends or family for ideas.

Describe one thing you have done to make a new friend and get someone to like you.

_____

_____

Check off and describe each skill that you used.

____Proximity   ____Similarity   ____Conversation skills   ____Expressed liking

_____

_____

Describe any efforts you made to join a conversational group. _____

_____

Describe any efforts you made to use your conversation skills with others. _____

_____

How effective was the interaction? _____

Mindfulness of Others

Due Date: _____   Name: _____ Week Starting: _____

Fill out this sheet whenever you practice mindfulness of others and whenever you have an opportunity to practice even if you don't (or almost don't) do anything to practice. Write on the back of this sheet if you need more room.

Check off any of the following that you practiced:

❑ Paid attention with interest and curiosity to others around me.
❑ Let go of a focus on myself, and focused on the people I was with.
❑ Noticed judgmental thoughts about others and let them go.
❑ Stayed in the present (instead of planning what I would say next) and listened.
❑ Put my entire attention on the other person and did not multitask.
❑ Gave up clinging to being right.
❑ Other: _____

❑ Described in a matter-of-fact way what I observed.
❑ Replaced judgmental descriptions with descriptive words.
❑ Described what I observed, instead of making assumptions and interpretations of others.
❑ Avoided questioning others' motives.
❑ Other: _____

❑ Threw myself into interactions with others.
❑ Went with the flow, rather than trying to control everything.
❑ Became one with the conversation I was in.
❑ Other: _____

Describe a situation where you practiced mindfulness of others in the last week. _____

_____

Who was the person you were with? _____

How exactly did you practice mindfulness? _____

What was the outcome? _____

_____

How did you feel afterward? _____

Did being mindful make a difference? If so, what? _____

_____

Ending Relationships

Due Date: _____ Name: _____ Week Starting: _____

Fill out this sheet to outline how to end an unwanted relationship when the relationship is not abusive. **If it is abusive, first call a local domestic violence hotline or the National Domestic Violence Hotline (1-800-799-7233).** Write on the back of this sheet if you need more room.

Relationship problem: Describe how the relationship is destructive or interfering with your life.

_____

_____

List Wise Mind pros and cons for ending the relationship.

Pros: _____

_____

Cons: _____

_____

Script Ideas for DEAR MAN, GIVE FAST to End a Relationship

1. **<u>D</u>escribe** the relationship situation, or the problem that is the core reason you want to end the relationship.

2. **<u>E</u>xpress** feelings/opinions about why the relationship needs to end for you.

3. **<u>A</u>ssert** in your decision to end the relationship directly (circle the part you will use later in "broken record" to stay mindful if you need it).

4. **<u>R</u>einforcing** comments to make about positive outcomes for both of you once the relationship is ended.

*(**continued on next page**)*

From *DBT Skills Training Handouts and Worksheets, Second Edition* by Marsha M. Linehan. Copyright 2015 by Marsha M. Linehan. Permission to photocopy this worksheet is granted to purchasers of this book for personal use only (see copyright page for details). Purchasers may download a larger version of this worksheet from *www.guilford.com/dbt-worksheets*.

5. **Mindful** and **Appearing confident** comments to make about how and when to end (if needed).

6. **Negotiating** comments to make, plus **turn-the-table** comments to avoid getting off track and responding to insults or diversions (if needed).

7. **Validating** comments about the other person's wishes, feelings, or history of the relationship.

8. **Easy manner** comments.

9. **Fair** comments.

Check off **opposite actions for love** you have been doing:

❑ 1. Reminded myself why love is not justified.

❑ 2. Did the opposite of loving urges.

❑ 3. Avoided contact with reminders of loved one.

❑ 4. Other: _____

Worksheets for Walking
the Middle Path

Practicing Dialectics

Due Date: _____   Name: _____   Week Starting: _____

Describe two situations that prompted you to practice dialectics.

SITUATION 1

Situation (who, what, when, where):

❑ Looked at both sides ❑ Stayed aware of my connection ❑ Embraced change ❑ Remembered that I affect others and others affect me	At left, check the skills you used, and describe here.

Describe experience of using the skill:

Check if practicing this dialectical skill has influenced any of the following, *even a little bit:*

____Reduced suffering   ____Increased happiness   ____Reduced friction with others
____Decreased reactivity   ____Increased wisdom   ____Improved relationship
____Increased connection   ____Increased sense of personal validity
____Other outcome: _____

SITUATION 2

Situation (who, what, when, where):

❑ Looked at both sides ❑ Stayed aware of my connection ❑ Embraced change ❑ Remembered that I affect others and others affect me	At left, check the skills you used, and describe here.

Describe experience of using the skill:

Check if practicing this dialectical skill has influenced any of the following, *even a little bit:*

____Reduced suffering   ____Increased happiness   ____Reduced friction with others
____Decreased reactivity   ____Increased wisdom   ____Improved relationship
____Increased connection   ____Increased sense of personal validity
____Other outcome: _____

Dialectics Checklist

Due Date: _____ Name: _____ Week Starting: _____

Everyday dialectical practice: Check off dialectical practice exercises each time you do one. For each skill you practice, give it a rating to indicate how effective that skill was in helping you reach your personal and interpersonal goals. Rate from a low of 1 (not at all effective) to a high of 5 (very effective).

Rating (1–5)

Looked at both sides:

▢▢▢▢ 1. Asked Wise Mind: "What am I missing?" ____

▢▢▢▢ 2. Looked for the kernel of truth in another person's side. ____

▢▢▢▢ 3. Stayed away from extremes (such as "always" or never"), and instead thought ____
or said: _____
_____

▢▢▢▢ 4. Balanced opposites in my life: ▢ Validated both myself and a person ____
I disagreed with ▢ Accepted reality and tried to change it ▢ Stayed
attached and also let go ▢ Other (describe): _____

▢▢▢▢ 5. Made lemonade out of lemons (describe): _____ ____
_____

▢▢▢▢ 6. Embraced confusion (describe): _____ ____

▢▢▢▢ 7. Played devil's advocate by arguing both my side and also the other side ____
(describe): _____
_____

▢▢▢▢ 8. Used a metaphor or story to describe my own point of view (describe): _____ ____
_____

▢▢▢▢ 9. Did 3-minute Wise Mind to slow down "doing mind" in my everyday life. ____

▢▢▢▢ 10. Other (describe): _____ ____

Stayed aware of my connection:

▢▢▢▢ 11. Treated others as I want to be treated (describe): _____ ____

▢▢▢▢ 12. Looked for similarities between myself and others (describe): _____ ____

▢▢▢▢ 13. Noticed the physical connections between all things (describe): _____ ____

▢▢▢▢ 14. Other (describe): _____ ____

Embraced change:

▢▢▢▢ 15. Practiced radical acceptance of change (describe): _____ ____

▢▢▢▢ 16. Purposely made changes in small ways to get used to change (describe): ___ ____
_____

▢▢▢▢ 17. Other (describe): _____ ____

Remembered that change is transactional:

▢▢▢▢ 18. Paid attention to my effect on others (describe): _____ ____

▢▢▢▢ 19. Paid attention to effect of others on me (describe): _____ ____

▢▢▢▢ 20. Practiced letting go of blame (describe): _____ ____

▢▢▢▢ 21. Reminded myself that all things, including all behaviors, are caused ____

▢▢▢▢ 22. Other (describe): _____ ____

Noticing When You're Not Dialectical

Due Date: _____ Name: _____ Week Starting: _____

Identify a time this week when you *did not use* your dialectical skills. Briefly describe the situation (who, what, when).

SITUATION 1

Situation (who, what, when, where):

❏ Looked at both sides
❏ Stayed aware of my connection
❏ Embraced change
❏ Remembered that I affect others and others affect me

At left, check the skills you needed but did not use, and describe here the experience of not using the skill.

What would you do differently next time?

Check if *not* practicing dialectical skills has influenced any of the following, *even a little bit:*

____Increased suffering   ____Decreased happiness   ____Increased friction with others
____Increased reactivity   ____Decreased wisdom   ____Harmed relationship
____Decreased connection   ____Other outcome: _____

SITUATION 2

Situation (who, what, when, where):

❏ Looked at both sides
❏ Stayed aware of my connection
❏ Embraced change
❏ Remembered that I affect others and others affect me

At left, check the skills you needed but did not use, and describe here the experience of not using the skill.

What would you do differently next time?

Check if *not* practicing dialectical skills has influenced any of the following, *even a little bit:*

____Increased suffering   ____Decreased happiness   ____Increased friction with others
____Increased reactivity   ____Decreased wisdom   ____Harmed relationship
____Decreased connection   ____Other outcome: _____

Validating Others

Due Date: _____   Name: _____   Week Starting: _____

Fill out this sheet whenever you practice your validation skills and whenever you have an opportunity to practice even if you don't (or almost don't) do anything to practice. Write on the back of this sheet if you need more room.

Check off types of validation that you practiced (on purpose) with others:

❑ 1. Paid attention.
❑ 2. Reflected back what was said or done, remaining open to correction.
❑ 3. Was sensitive to what was unsaid.

❑ 4. Expressed how what was felt, done, or said made sense, given the causes.
❑ 5. Acknowledged and acted on what was valid.
❑ 6. Acted authentically and as an equal.

List one invalidating and two validating statements made to others.

1. _____

2. _____

3. _____

Describe a situation where you were nonjudgmental of someone in the past week.

_____

_____

_____

Describe a situation where you used validation in the past week.

_____

_____

_____

Who was the person you validated? _____

What exactly did you do or say to validate the person? _____

_____

_____

What was the outcome? _____

_____

_____

How did you feel afterward? _____

Would you say or do something differently next time? If so, what? _____

_____

Self-Validation and Self-Respect

Due Date: _____ Name: _____ Week Starting: _____

Fill out this sheet whenever you practice your self-validation skills and whenever you have an opportunity to practice even if you don't (or almost don't) do anything to practice. Write on the back of this sheet if you need more room.

List one self-invalidating and two self-validating statements you made.

1. _____

2. _____

3. _____

Describe a situation where you felt invalidated in the past week: _____

_____

_____

Check each strategy you used during the week:

❑ Checked *all* the facts to see if my responses are valid or invalid.

❑ Checked it out with someone I could trust to validate the valid.

❑ Acknowledged when my responses didn't make sense and were not valid.

❑ Worked to change invalid thinking, comments, or actions. (Stopped blaming.)

❑ Dropped judgmental self-statements. (Practiced opposite action.)

❑ Reminded myself that all behavior is caused and that I am doing my best.

❑ Was compassionate toward myself. Practiced self-soothing.

❑ Admitted that it hurts to be invalidated by others, even if they are right.

❑ Acknowledged when my reactions make sense and are valid in a situation.

❑ Remembered that being invalidated, even when my response is actually valid, is rarely a complete catastrophe.

❑ Described my experiences and actions in a supportive environment.

❑ Grieved traumatic invalidation in my life and the harm it has created.

❑ Practiced radical acceptance of the invalidating person(s) in my life.

❑ **What was the outcome?** _____

_____

_____

Changing Behavior with Reinforcement

Due Date: _____ Name: _____ Week Starting: _____

Fill out this sheet whenever you try to increase your own or someone else's behavior with reinforcement. Look for opportunities (since they occur all the time) to reinforce behavior. Write on the back of this sheet if you need more room.

1. In advance, identify the behavior you want to increase and the reinforcer you will use.

    a. For yourself:

        Behavior to increase: _____

        Reinforcer: _____

    b. For someone else:

        Behavior to increase: _____

        Reinforcer: _____

2. Describe the situation(s) where you used reinforcement.

    a. For yourself: _____

    b. For someone else: _____

3. What was the outcome? What did you observe?

    a. For yourself: _____

    _____

    _____

    _____

    b. For someone else: _____

    _____

    _____

4. How did you feel afterward? _____

_____

5. Would you say or do something differently next time? If so, what? _____

_____

Changing Behavior by Extinguishing or Punishing It

Due Date: _____   Name: _____   Week Starting: _____

Fill out this sheet whenever you try to increase your own or someone else's behavior with reinforcement. Look for opportunities (since they occur all the time) to reinforce behavior. Write on the back of this sheet if you need more room.

1. **In advance, identify the behavior you want to decrease, and decide whether you will extinguish it by eliminating a reinforcer or stop it with punishment.** (Skip the one you are not using.)

   If you are using punishment, identify the consequence. Also decide the new alternative behavior to reinforce, and the reinforcer to use to increase it to replace the behavior you are decreasing.

   a. For yourself:

   Behavior to decrease: _____

   Reinforcer to remove: _____

   Punishing consequence to add: _____

   New behavior and reinforcer: _____

   b. For someone else:

   Behavior to decrease: _____

   Reinforcer to remove: _____

   Punishing consequence to add: _____

   New behavior and reinforcer: _____

2. **Describe the situation(s) where you used extinction or punishment.** (Circle which you use.)

   a. For yourself: _____

   b. For someone else: _____

3. **What was the outcome? What did you observe?**

   a. For yourself: _____

   _____

   b. For someone else: _____

   _____

4. **How did you feel afterward?** _____

   _____

5. **Would you do something differently next time? If so, what?** _____

   _____

EMOTION
REGULATION SKILLS

Introduction to Handouts and Worksheets

The goal of emotion regulation is to reduce emotional suffering. The goal is not to get rid of emotions; emotions have important functions in our lives. Emotion regulation skills help you to change emotions that you (not other people) want to change, or to reduce the intensity of your emotions. Emotion regulation skills can also reduce your vulnerability to becoming extremely or painfully emotional and increase your emotional resilience. Emotion regulation requires use of mindfulness skills, particularly nonjudgmental observation and description of your own current emotions. You have to know what an emotion is and what it does for you before you can effectively regulate it.

There are four sets of handouts and worksheets for emotion regulation skills: **Understanding and Naming Emotions; Changing Emotional Responses; Reducing Vulnerability to Emotion Mind;** and **Managing Really Difficult Emotions.** There is also one introductory handout–worksheet pair:

• **Emotion Regulation Handout 1: Goals of Emotion Regulation.** This handout briefly outlines the goals of the skills taught in this module. It can be used with **Emotion Regulation Worksheet 1: Pros and Cons of Changing Emotions.**

Understanding and Naming Emotions

• **Emotion Regulation Handout 2: Overview: Understanding and Naming Emotions.** It is difficult to manage your emotions when you do not understand how emotions work. Knowledge is power. This handout overviews the skills covered in this section.

• **Emotion Regulation Handout 3: What Emotions Do for You.** There are reasons why humans (and many other animals) have emotions. They have three important functions and we need them. If you have been through the Emotion Regulation module at least once, the following worksheets may be useful. If you are learning emotion regulation skills for the first time, skip these worksheets until later.

• **Emotion Regulation Worksheet 2: Figuring Out What My Emotions Are Doing for Me.** This worksheet can be used with Emotion Regulation Handout 3. **Emotion Regulation Worksheet 2a: Example: Figuring Out What My Emotions Are Doing for Me** is a filled-in example of Worksheet 2.

• **Emotion Regulation Worksheet 2b: Emotion Diary.** This is a worksheet in a different format that can also be used with Handout 3, to identify how your emotions are functioning over time. **Emotion Regulation Worksheet 2c: Example: Emotion Diary** is a filled-in example of Worksheet 2c.

• **Emotion Regulation Handout 4: What Makes It Hard to Regulate Your Emotions.** Regulating emotions is very hard. Biology, lack of skills, reinforcing consequences, moodiness, mental overload, and emotion myths can each make regulating emotions difficult.

• **Emotion Regulation Handout 4a: Myths about Emotions.** Do you believe any of the myths on this handout? Use **Emotion Regulation Worksheet 3: Myths about Emotions** to challenge emotion myths that may be getting in your way.

• **Emotion Regulation Handout 5: A Model for Describing Emotions.** Emotions are complex and consist of several parts that happen at the same time. Changing any part of this emotional response system can change the entire response. Knowing the parts of an emotion can help you change the emotion. This handout shows these parts in some detail.

• **Emotion Regulation Handout 6: Ways to Describe Emotion.** This long handout lists the typical parts for 10 specific emotions: anger, disgust, envy, fear, happiness, jealousy, love, sadness, shame, and guilt. The sections within each emotion on this handout generally match the parts illustrated in Emotion Regulation Handout 5. The emotion features listed in Handout 6 are not necessary to each emotion, and these features may differ from person to person.

Record your practice on either **Emotion Regulation Worksheet 4 or 4a: Observing and Describing Emotions.** These two worksheets differ in format, but ask for exactly the same information. Worksheet 4 is in the same flow chart format as the models for describing emotion (Handout 5). Worksheet 4a is in a list format. Refer to Handout 6 for ideas if you have trouble describing or identifying your emotion. Note that the "Prompting Event" consists of only the few moments immediately before the emotion fires up. The history, or story, leading up to the prompting event goes under "Vulnerability Factors." Don't forget to put in physical illness or pain, alcohol and drug use, lack of sleep, over- or undereating, and stressful events in the 24 hours before the prompting event. To rate the intensity of an emotion, use a 0–100 scale in which 0 is no emotion and 100 is the most extreme emotion.

Changing Emotional Responses

• **Emotion Regulation Handout 7: Overview: Changing Emotional Responses.** This handout introduces the three skills for changing emotions: checking the facts, opposite action, and problem solving.

• **Emotion Regulation Handout 8: Checking the Facts.** We often react to our thoughts and interpretations of an event rather than to the facts of the event. Changing our beliefs, assumptions, and interpretations of events to fit the facts can change our emotional reactions. Use **Emotion Regulation Worksheet 5: Checking the Facts** to record practice of this skill. Notice that this worksheet has spaces for you to write down descriptions of the situation (Step 2) and descriptions of the thoughts and interpretations that are likely to be setting off the emotion (Step 3). It then provides additional space in each step for you to check the facts—that is, to consider alternative descriptions, as well as alternative interpretations of the situation. At the top of the worksheet, rate the intensity of your emotion (0 = no emotion, 100 = maximum intensity) before checking the facts and then after checking the facts.

• **Emotion Regulation Handout 8a: Examples of Emotions That Fit the Facts.** When unwanted emotions fit the facts, then checking the facts will not change the emotion. This handout lists emotions together with examples of facts that fit them. To change these emotions, either opposite action or problem solving should be used.

• **Emotion Regulation Handout 9: Opposite Action and Problem Solving: Deciding Which to Use.** When emotions fit the facts, changing the situation through problem solving can be the most effective way to change the emotion. At other times, changing how you feel about the situation through opposite action is the best course of action. The flow chart on this handout can help you figure out what skill to use to change frequent but unwanted emotions. Use **Emotion Regulation Worksheet 6: Figuring Out How to Change Unwanted Emotions** to work out which skill to use. This worksheet has the same flow chart format as Handout 9.

• **Emotion Regulation Handout 10: Opposite Action** and **Emotion Regulation Handout 11: Figuring Out Opposite Action.** Opposite action is acting opposite to your emotional urge to do or say something. Opposite action is an effective way to change or reduce unwanted emotions. The action urge is one of the parts of an emotion (see Emotion Regulation Handout 5), and each emotion has a typical action urge (see Emotion Regulation Handout 6). Handout 10 lists the steps for how to do opposite action. Handout 11 is a guide for identifying opposite actions for nine specific emotions. The opposite actions on Handout 11 are, however, only suggestions. It's important to identify your own action urges and figure out actions opposite to those urges. To record your practice of opposite action, use **Emotion Regulation Worksheet 7: Opposite Action to Change Emotions.** The "Before" and "After" spaces are for rating the emotion's intensity before practicing opposite action and afterward. When you are analyzing whether the emotion is justified (i.e., whether it fits the facts), focus on the emotion's prompting event.

• **Emotion Regulation Handout 12: Problem Solving.** When an emotion fits the facts of the situation, avoiding or changing the situation may be the best way to change the emotion. Problem solving is the first step in changing difficult situations. The steps of problem solving are listed on this handout. To record your practice of this skill, use **Emotion Regulation Worksheet 8: Problem Solving to Change Emotions.** Filling out this worksheet can be helpful in figuring out the problem and how to solve it, but actually solving the problem (i.e., taking Steps 6 and 7 on the worksheet) is most important to changing emotions. Rate the intensity of the emotion (0–100) both before and after implementing a solution.

• **Emotion Regulation Handout 13: Reviewing Opposite Action and Problem Solving.** It's important to know not only when to use opposite action or problem solving but also to know how these two skills differ in actual practice. In its first column, Handout 13 summarizes "justifying events" (i.e., situations that fit the facts) for each basic emotion. The second column lists examples of opposite actions. This skill is used for unjustified emotions or justified emotions when acting on that emotion would be ineffective. The third column lists examples of acting on the urge of a justified emotion, such as through problem solving or avoidance. Notice that the justifying events on Handout 13 are the same as the prompting events in Emotion Regulation Handout 6: Ways to Describe Emotions. Both justifying events and opposite actions on Handout 13 are shorthand versions of Emotion Regulation Handout 11: Figuring Out Opposite Actions.

Reducing Vulnerability to Emotion Mind

• **Emotion Regulation Handout 14: Overview: Reducing Vulnerability to Emotion Mind—Building a Live Worth Living.** Emotional distress and anguish can be reduced by decreasing factors that make you vulnerable to negative emotions and moods. This handout is an overview of the skills in this section, which can be remembered with the term ABC PLEASE: Accumulate positive emotions; Build mastery; Cope ahead of time with emotional situations; and take care of your mind by taking care of your body (the PLEASE skills). **Emotion Regulation Worksheet 9: Steps for Reducing Vulnerability to Emotion Mind** is a summary worksheet for all the ABC PLEASE skills and can be used for practicing any or all of the skills.

• **Emotion Regulation Handout 15: Accumulating Positive Emotions: Short Term** and **Emotion Regulation Handout 16: Pleasant Events List.** Handout 15 is an overview of building positive experiences now by increasing pleasant events and experiences. Handout 16 is a list of pleasant events. Which events on this list would you find pleasant? Do as many of these things as you can that would make you happy or joyful, even if they seem only a little effective for this at first. **Emotion Regulation Worksheet 10: Pleasant Events Diary** is designed to be filled out daily. Write out your plans for the week, and then write down what you actually did. Rate how mindful you were to the event (i.e., how focused and in the moment you were, how much you participated). Finally, how unmindful were you of worries, and how pleasant was the experience? Emotion Regulation Worksheets 9 and 13 also have brief sections for tracking pleasant events, along with other ABC PLEASE skills.

• **Emotion Regulation Handout 17: Accumulating Positive Emotions: Long Term,** and **Emotion Regulation Handout 18: Values and Priorities List.** It is hard to be happy without a life experienced as worth living. Building such a life requires attention to your own values and life priorities, and it can take time, patience, and persistence. Handout 17 breaks down the process of building a life worth living into seven steps. Handout 18 helps with Step 2, "Identify values that are important to you," by listing 58 specific values grouped into 13 categories. You can choose a general value, specific values, a combination, or values not on the list.

• **Emotion Regulation Worksheets 11** and **11a: Getting from Values to Specific Action Steps.** Both these worksheets are designed to help you work out what steps are needed to build a life you want to live. Worksheet 11 provides more space and also emphasizes attending to relationships as a value.

• **Emotion Regulation Worksheet 11b: Diary of Daily Actions on Values and Priorities.** This is an advanced worksheet for keeping track of actions taken across different life goals and values. It is intended for those already experienced with DBT skills, rather than those beginning skills training.

• **Emotion Regulation Handout 19: Build Mastery and Cope Ahead.** Feeling competent and adequately prepared for difficult situations reduces vulnerability to negative emotions and increases skillful behavior. This handout covers steps for two skills: build mastery and cope ahead of emotional situations. Use **Emotion Regulation Worksheet 12: Build Mastery and Cope Ahead** to schedule activities to build a sense of accomplishment and then report on what you actually did. There is also space to report on two practices of "cope ahead."

• **Emotion Regulation Worksheet 13: Putting ABC Skills Together Day by Day.** This worksheet has a brief section for tracking <u>A</u>ccumulate positive emotions, <u>B</u>uild mastery, and <u>C</u>ope ahead.

• **Emotion Regulation Handout 20: Taking Care of Your Mind by Taking Care of Your Body.** An out-of-balance body increases vulnerability to negative emotions and emotion mind. Taking care of your body increases emotional resilience. The acronym PLEASE covers treating <u>P</u>hysica<u>L</u> illness, balancing <u>E</u>ating, avoiding mood-<u>A</u>ltering substances, balancing <u>S</u>leep, and getting <u>E</u>xercise. **Emotion Regulation Worksheet 14: Practicing PLEASE Skills** can be used to record practice during the week. There is a row for each day; record how you practiced PLEASE skills that day. At the bottom of each column is a space to check whether the specific skill was helpful over the week.

• **Emotion Regulation Handout 20a: Nightmare Protocol, Step by Step.** Follow the steps on this handout if nightmares disturb your sleep. Fill out **Emotion Regulation Worksheet 14a: Target Nightmare Experience Form** to follow the protocol on Handout 20a. Note that this worksheet consists of three forms: the Target Nightmare Experience Form, the Changed Dream Experience Form, and the Dream

Rehearsal and Relaxation Record. Some people find it easier to start with the second form.

• **Emotion Regulation Handout 20b: Sleep Hygiene Protocol.** When worries keep you from sleeping, try the steps on this handout. Use **Emotion Regulation Worksheet 14b: Sleep Hygiene Practice Sheet** to record your experience.

Managing Really Difficult Emotions

• **Emotion Regulation Handout 21: Overview: Managing Really Difficult Emotions.** At times the intensity of negative emotions can be so high that special skills are necessary to manage them. This handout is an overview of these skills.

• **Emotion Regulation Handout 22: Mindfulness of Current Emotions: Letting Go of Emotional Suffering.** Mindfulness of current emotions means observing, describing, and "allowing" emotions without judging them or trying to change, block, or distract from them. Avoiding or suppressing emotion increases suffering. Mindfulness of current emotions is the path to emotional freedom. It is a critical skill underpinning many, if not most, skills in DBT. Avoiding emotions interferes with using almost every other skill in this module. To record practice of this skill, use **Emotion Regulation Worksheet 15: Mindfulness of Current Emotions.** It allows you to check off what skills you used. If you have trouble identifying the emotion you are feeling, review Emotion Regulation Handout 6: Ways to Describe Emotions. On Worksheet 15, remember to rate the intensity of the emotion before and after you practice mindfulness of current emotions.

• **Emotion Regulation Handout 23: Managing Extreme Emotions.** When your emotional arousal is very high, your ability to use your skills breaks down. Knowing your skills breakdown point is important; it signals the need to use crisis survival skills (which are taught in the Distress Tolerance module) first. This handout teaches you how to identify your skills breakdown point.

• **Emotion Regulation Handout 24: Troubleshooting Emotion Regulation Skills.** When one or more of the emotion regulation skills do not seem to work, do not give up on the skills. Instead, troubleshoot how they are being applied. This handout helps you figure out what is interfering with your efforts to manage difficult or ineffective emotions. You can also use **Emotion Regulation Worksheet 16: Troubleshooting Emotion Regulation Skills,** which goes over much of the same information.

Emotion
Regulation Handouts

Goals of Emotion Regulation

UNDERSTAND AND NAME YOUR OWN EMOTIONS

❑ Identify (observe and describe) your emotions.

❑ Know what emotions do for you.

❑ Other: _____

DECREASE THE FREQUENCY OF UNWANTED EMOTIONS

❑ Stop unwanted emotions from starting in the first place.

❑ Change unwanted emotions once they start.

❑ Other: _____

DECREASE EMOTIONAL VULNERABILITY

❑ Decrease vulnerability to emotion mind.

❑ Increase resilience, your ability to cope with difficult things and positive emotions.

❑ Other: _____

DECREASE EMOTIONAL SUFFERING

❑ Reduce suffering when painful emotions overcome you.

❑ Manage extreme emotions so that you don't make things worse.

❑ Other: _____

··

*Handouts for Understanding
and Naming Emotions*

··

Overview:
Understanding and Naming Emotions

WHAT EMOTIONS DO FOR YOU

There are reasons why we have emotions.

We need them!

FACTORS THAT MAKE
REGULATING EMOTIONS HARD

Lack of skills, reinforcing consequences, moodiness, rumination/worrying, myths about emotions, and biology can interfere with changing emotions.

A MODEL FOR DESCRIBING EMOTIONS

Emotions are complex responses.

Changing any part of the system can change the entire response.

WAYS TO DESCRIBE EMOTIONS

Learning to observe, describe, and name your emotion can help you regulate your emotions.

What Emotions Do for You

EMOTIONS MOTIVATE (AND ORGANIZE) US FOR ACTION

- Emotions motivate our behavior. Emotions prepare us for action.
  The action urge of specific emotions is often "hard-wired" in biology.

- Emotions save time in getting us to act in important situations.
  Emotions can be especially important when we don't have time to think things through.

- Strong emotions help us overcome obstacles—in our minds and in the environment.

EMOTIONS COMMUNICATE TO (AND INFLUENCE) OTHERS

- Facial expressions are hard-wired aspects of emotions.
  Facial expressions communicate faster than words.

- Our body language and voice tone can also be hard-wired.
  Like it or not, they also communicate our emotions to others.

- When it is important to communicate to others, or send them a message,
  it can be very hard to change our emotions.

- Whether we intend it or not, our communication of emotions influences others.

EMOTIONS COMMUNICATE TO OURSELVES

- Emotional reactions can give us important information about a situation.
  Emotions can be signals or alarms that something is happening.

- Gut feelings can be like intuition—a response to something important about the situation.
  This can be helpful if our emotions get us to check out the facts.

- **Caution:** Sometimes we treat emotions as if they are facts about the world: The stronger
  the emotion, the stronger our belief that the emotion is based on fact. (Examples: "If I feel
  unsure, I am incompetent," "If I get lonely when left alone, I shouldn't be left alone," "If I feel
  confident about something, it is right," "If I'm afraid, there must be danger," "I love him, so
  he must be OK.")

- If we assume that our emotions represent facts about the world, we may use them to justify
  our thoughts or our actions. This can be trouble if our emotions get us to ignore the facts.

What Makes It Hard to Regulate Your Emotions

BIOLOGY

❏ Biological factors can make emotion regulation harder.

LACK OF SKILL

❏ You don't know what to do to regulate your emotions.

REINFORCEMENT OF EMOTIONAL BEHAVIOR

❏ Your environment reinforces you when you are highly emotional.

MOODINESS

❏ Your current mood controls what you do instead of your Wise Mind.
❏ You don't really want to put in time and effort to regulate your emotions.

EMOTIONAL OVERLOAD

❏ High emotional arousal causes you to reach a skills breakdown point. You can't follow skills instructions or figure out what to do.

EMOTION MYTHS

❏ Myths (e.g., mistaken beliefs) about emotions get in the way of your ability to regulate emotions.
   ❏ Myths that emotions are bad or weak lead to avoiding emotions.
   ❏ Myths that extreme emotions are necessary or are part of who you are keep you from trying to regulate your emotions.

Myths about Emotions

1. There is a right way to feel in every situation.
   Challenge: _____

2. Letting others know that I am feeling bad is a weakness.
   Challenge: _____

3. Negative feelings are bad and destructive.
   Challenge: _____

4. Being emotional means being out of control.
   Challenge: _____

5. Some emotions are stupid.
   Challenge: _____

6. All painful emotions are a result of a bad attitude.
   Challenge: _____

7. If others don't approve of my feelings, I obviously shouldn't feel the way I do.
   Challenge: _____

8. Other people are the best judges of how I am feeling.
   Challenge: _____

9. Painful emotions are not important and should be ignored.
   Challenge: _____

10. Extreme emotions get you a lot further than trying to regulate your emotions.
    Challenge: _____

11. Creativity requires intense, often out-of-control emotions.
    Challenge: _____

12. Drama is cool.
    Challenge: _____

13. It is inauthentic to try to change my emotions.
    Challenge: _____

14. Emotional truth is what counts, not factual truth.
    Challenge: _____

15. People should do whatever they feel like doing.
    Challenge: _____

16. Acting on your emotions is the mark of a truly free individual.
    Challenge: _____

17. My emotions are who I am.
    Challenge: _____

18. My emotions are why people love me.
    Challenge: _____

19. Emotions can just happen for no reason.
    Challenge: _____

20. Emotions should always be trusted.
    Challenge: _____

21. Other myth: _____

    Challenge: _____

Model for Describing Emotions

Emotion Name

Awareness

Expressions

Face and Body Language
(facial expression, posture, gestures, skin color)

Words
(what you say)

Actions
(your behavior)

Biological Changes

Brain changes
(neural firing)

Nervous system changes
(internal body changes
that affect muscles
and autonomic system
firing—blood vessels,
heart rate, temperature)

Experiences

Body sensations (feelings)

Action urges

Preexisting Vulnerability Factors

Interpretation
(Thoughts/beliefs about prompting event)

Attention/Awareness

Prompting Event

Attention/Awareness

Prompting Event 2

Secondary Emotions

Aftereffects

Ways to Describe Emotions

ANGER WORDS

anger	bitterness	fury	indignation	vengefulness
aggravation	exasperation	grouchiness	irritation	wrath
agitation	ferocity	grumpiness	outrage	
annoyance	frustration	hostility	rage	

Prompting Events for Feeling Anger

- Having an important goal blocked.
- You or someone you care about being attacked or threatened by others.
- Losing power, status, or respect.
- Not having things turn out as expected.
- Physical or emotional pain.
- Other: _____

Interpretations of Events That Prompt Feelings of Anger

- Believing that you have been treated unfairly.
- Blaming.
- Believing that important goals are being blocked or stopped.
- Believing that things "should" be different than they are.
- Rigidly thinking, "I'm right."
- Judging that the situation is illegitimate or wrong.
- Ruminating about the event that set off the anger in the first place.
- Other: _____

Biological Changes and Experiences of Anger

- Muscles tightening.
- Teeth clamping together.
- Hands clenching.
- Feeling your face flush or get hot.
- Feeling like you are going to explode.
- Being unable to stop tears.
- Wanting to hit someone, bang the wall, throw something, blow up.
- Wanting to hurt someone.
- Other: _____

Expressions and Actions of Anger

- Physically or verbally attacking.
- Making aggressive or threatening gestures.
- Pounding, throwing things, breaking things.
- Walking heavily, stomping, slamming doors.
- Walking out.
- Using a loud, quarrelsome, or sarcastic voice.
- Using obscenities or swearing.
- Criticizing or complaining.
- Clenching your hands or fists.
- Frowning, not smiling, mean expression.
- Brooding or withdrawing from others.
- Crying.
- Grinning.
- A red or flushed face.
- Other: _____

Aftereffects of Anger

- Narrowing of attention.
- Attending only to the situation that's making you angry.
- Ruminating about the situation making you angry or about situations in the past.
- Imagining future situations that will make you angry.
- Depersonalization, dissociative experiences, numbness.
- Other: _____

(*continued on next page*)

Note. Adapted from Table 3 in Shaver, P., Schwartz, J., Kirson, D., & O'Connor, C. (1987). Emotion knowledge: Further exploration of a proto-type approach. *Journal of Personality and Social Psychology, 52*(6), 1061–1086. Copyright 1987 by the American Psychological Association. Adapted by permission.

DISGUST WORDS

disgust	aversion	dislike	distaste	repugnance	resentment	sickened
abhorrence	condescension	derision	hate	repelled	revolted	spite
antipathy	contempt	disdain	loathing	repulsion	scorn	vile

Prompting Events for Feeling Disgust

- Seeing/smelling human or animal waste products.
- Having a person or an animal that is dirty, slimy, or unclean come close to you.
- Tasting something or being forced to swallow something you really don't want.
- Seeing or being near a dead body.
- Touching items worn or owned by a stranger, dead person, or disliked person.
- Observing or hearing about a person who grovels or who strips another person of dignity.
- Seeing blood; getting blood drawn.
- Observing or hearing about a person acting with extreme hypocrisy/fawning.
- Observing or hearing about betrayal, child abuse, racism, or other types of cruelty.
- Being forced to watch something that deeply violates your own Wise Mind values.
- Being confronted with someone who is deeply violating your own Wise Mind values.
- Being forced to engage in or watch unwanted sexual contact.
- Other: _____

Interpretations of Events That Prompt Feelings of Disgust

- Believing that:
  - You are swallowing something toxic.
  - Your skin or your mind is being contaminated.
  - Your own body or body parts are ugly.
  - Others are evil or the "scum" of the earth, or that they disrespect authority or the group.
- Disapproving of/feeling morally superior to another.
- Extreme disapproval of yourself or your own feelings, thoughts, or behaviors.
- Judging that a person is deeply immoral or has sinned or violated the natural order of things.
- Judging someone's body as extremely ugly.
- Other: _____

Biological Changes and Experiences of Disgust

- Feelings of nausea; sick feeling.
- Urge to vomit, vomiting, gagging, choking.
- Having a lump in your throat.
- Aversion to drinking or eating.
- Intense urge to destroy or get rid of something.
- Urge to take a shower.
- Urge to run away or push away.
- Feeling contaminated, dirty, unclean.
- Feeling mentally polluted.
- Fainting.
- Other: _____

Expressions and Actions of Disgust

- Vomiting, spitting out.
- Closing your eyes, looking away.
- Washing, scrubbing, taking a bath.
- Changing your clothes; cleaning spaces.
- Avoiding eating or drinking.
- Pushing or kicking away; running away.
- Treating with disdain or disrespect.
- Stepping over; crowding another person out.
- Physically attacking causes of your disgust.
- Using obscenities or cursing.
- Clenching your hands or fists.
- Frowning, or not smiling.
- Mean or unpleasant facial expression.
- Speaking with a sarcastic voice tone.
- Nose and top lip tightened up; smirking.
- Other: _____

Aftereffects of Disgust

- Narrowing of attention.
- Ruminating about the situation that's making you feel disgusted.
- Becoming hypersensitive to dirt.
- Other: _____

*(**continued on next page**)*

215

ENVY WORDS

envy	craving	displeased	greed	pettiness
bitterness	discontented	dissatisfied	"green-eyed"	resentment
covetous	disgruntled	down-hearted	longing	wishful

Prompting Events for Feeling Envy

- Someone has something you really want or need but don't or can't have.
- You are not part of the "in" crowd.
- Someone appears to have everything.
- You are alone while others are having fun.
- Someone else gets credit for what you've done.
- Someone gets positive recognition for something and you don't.
- Others get something you really want and you don't get it.
- Being around people who have more than you have.
- Someone you are competing with is more successful than you in an area important to you.
- Other: _____

Interpretations of Events That Prompt Feelings of Envy

- Thinking you deserve what others have.
- Thinking others have more than you.
- Thinking about how unfair it is that you have such a bad lot in life compared to others.
- Thinking you have been treated unfairly by life.
- Thinking you are unlucky.
- Thinking you are inferior, a failure, or mediocre in comparison to others whom you want to be like.
- Comparing yourself to others who have more than you.
- Comparing yourself to people who have characteristics that you wish you had.
- Thinking you are unappreciated.
- Other: _____

Biological Changes and Experiences of Envy

- Muscles tightening.
- Teeth clamping together, mouth tightening.
- Feeling your face flush or get hot.
- Feeling rigidity in your body.
- Pain in the pit of the stomach.
- Having an urge to get even.
- Hating the other person.
- Wanting to hurt the people you envy.
- Wanting the person or people you envy to lose what they have, to have bad luck, or to be hurt.
- Feeling pleasure when others experience failure or lose what they have.
- Feeling unhappy if another person experiences some good luck.
- Feeling motivated to improve yourself.
- Other: _____

Expressions and Actions of Envy

- Doing everything you can to get what the other person has.
- Working a lot harder than you were to get what you want.
- Trying to improve yourself and your situation.
- Taking away or ruining what the other person has.
- Attacking or criticizing the other person.
- Doing something to get even.
- Doing something to make the other person fail or lose what he or she has.
- Saying mean things about the other person or making the person look bad to others.
- Trying to show the other person up, to look better than the other person.
- Avoiding persons who have what you want.
- Other: _____

Aftereffects of Envy

- Narrowing of attention.
- Attending only to what others have that you don't.
- Ruminating when others have had more than you.
- Discounting what you do have; not appreciating things you have or things others do for you.
- Ruminating about what you don't have.
- Making resolutions to change.
- Other: _____

(*continued on next page*)

FEAR WORDS

fear	dread	horror	nervousness	shock	uneasiness
anxiety	edginess	hysteria	overwhelmed	tenseness	worry
apprehension	fright	jumpiness	panic	terror	

Prompting Events for Feeling Fear

- Having your life, your health, or your well-being threatened.
- Being in the same situation (or a similar one) where you have been threatened or gotten hurt in the past, or where painful things have happened.
- Flashbacks.
- Being in situations where you have seen others threatened or be hurt.

- Silence.
- Being in a new or unfamiliar situation.
- Being alone (e.g., walking alone, being home alone, living alone).
- Being in the dark.
- Being in crowds.
- Leaving your home.
- Having to perform in front of others.
- Pursuing your dreams.
- Other: _____

Interpretations of Events That Prompt Feelings of Fear

- Believing that:
  - You might die, or you are going to die.
  - You might be hurt or harmed.
  - You might lose something valuable.
  - Someone might reject, criticize, or dislike you.
  - You will embarrass yourself.
  - Failure is possible; expecting to fail.

- Believing that:
  - You will not get help you want or need.
  - You might lose help you already have.
  - You might lose someone important.
  - You might lose something you want.
  - You are helpless or are losing a sense of control.
  - You are incompetent or are losing mastery.
- Other: _____

Biological Changes and Experiences of Fear

- Breathlessness.
- Fast heartbeat.
- Choking sensation, lump in throat.
- Muscles tensing, cramping.
- Clenching teeth.
- Urge to scream or call out.

- Feeling nauseated.
- Getting cold; feeling clammy.
- Feeling your hairs standing on end.
- Feeling of "butterflies" in stomach.
- Wanting to run away or avoid things.
- Other: _____

Expressions and Actions of Fear

- Fleeing, running away.
- Running or walking hurriedly.
- Hiding from or avoiding what you fear.
- Engaging in nervous, fearful talk.
- Pleading or crying for help.
- Talking less or becoming speechless.
- Screaming or yelling.
- Darting eyes or quickly looking around.
- Frozen stare.

- Talking yourself out of doing what you fear.
- Freezing, or trying not to move.
- Crying or whimpering.
- Shaking, quivering, or trembling.
- A shaky or trembling voice.
- Sweating or perspiring.
- Diarrhea, vomiting.
- Hair erect.
- Other: _____

Aftereffects of Fear

- Narrowing of attention.
- Being hypervigilant to threat.
- Losing your ability to focus or becoming disoriented or dazed.
- Losing control.

- Imagining the possibility of more loss or failure.
- Isolating yourself.
- Ruminating about other threatening times.
- Other: _____

(*continued on next page*)

HAPPINESS WORDS

happiness	satisfaction	joviality	exhilaration	ecstasy
joy	bliss	triumph	optimism	gladness
enjoyment	enthusiasm	contentment	zest	pride
relief	jolliness	excitement	eagerness	elation
amusement	thrill	jubilation	gaiety	glee
enthrallment	cheerfulness	zaniness	pleasure	rapture
hope	euphoria	delight	zeal	

Prompting Events for Feeling Happiness

- Receiving a wonderful surprise.
- Reality exceeding your expectations.
- Getting what you want.
- Getting something you have worked hard for or worried about.
- Things turning out better than you thought they would.
- Being successful at a task.
- Achieving a desirable outcome.
- Receiving esteem, respect, or praise.
- Receiving love, liking, or affection.
- Being accepted by others.
- Belonging somewhere or with someone or a group.
- Being with or in contact with people who love or like you.
- Having very pleasurable sensations.
- Doing things that create or bring to mind pleasurable sensations.
- Other: _____

Interpretations of Events That Prompt Feelings of Happiness

- Interpreting joyful events just as they are, without adding or subtracting.
- Other: _____

Biological Changes and Experiences of Happiness

- Feeling excited.
- Feeling physically energetic, active.
- Feeling like giggling or laughing.
- Feeling your face flush.
- Feeling calm all the way through.
- Urge to keep doing what is associated with happiness.
- Feeling at peace.
- Feeling open or expansive.
- Other: _____

Expressions and Actions of Happiness

- Smiling.
- Having a bright, glowing face.
- Being bouncy or bubbly.
- Communicating your good feelings.
- Sharing the feeling.
- Silliness.
- Hugging people.
- Jumping up and down.
- Saying positive things.
- Using an enthusiastic or excited voice.
- Being talkative or talking a lot.
- Other: _____

Aftereffects of Happiness

- Being courteous or friendly to others.
- Doing nice things for other people.
- Having a positive outlook; seeing the bright side.
- Having a high threshold for worry or annoyance.
- Remembering and imagining other times you have felt joyful.
- Expecting to feel joyful in the future.
- Other: _____

(*continued on next page*)

JEALOUSY WORDS

jealous	clutching	fear of losing someone/	rivalrous	wary
cautious	defensive	something	suspicious	watchful
clinging	mistrustful	possessive	self-protective	

Prompting Events for Feeling Jealous

- An important relationship is threatened or in danger of being lost.
- A potential competitor pays attention to someone you love.
- Someone:
  - Is threatening to take away important things in your life.
  - Goes out with the person you like.
  - Ignores you while talking to a friend of yours.
  - Is more attractive, outgoing, or self-confident than you.
- You are treated as unimportant by a person you want to be close to.
- Your partner tells you that he or she desires more time alone.
- Your partner appears to flirt with someone else.
- A person you are romantically involved with looks at someone else.
- You find the person you love is having an affair with someone else.
- Other: _____

Interpretations of Events That Prompt Feelings of Jealousy

- Believing that:
  - Your partner does not care for you any more.
  - You are nothing to your partner.
  - Your partner is going to leave you.
  - Your partner is behaving inappropriately.
  - You don't measure up to your peers.
  - I deserve more than what you are receiving.
- Believing that:
  - You were cheated.
  - No one cares about you.
  - Your rival is possessive and competitive.
  - Your rival is insecure.
  - Your rival is envious.
  - Other: _____

Biological Changes and Experiences of Jealousy

- Breathlessness.
- Fast heartbeat.
- Choking sensation, lump in throat.
- Muscles tensing.
- Teeth clenching.
- Becoming suspicious of others.
- Having injured pride.
- Feelings of rejection.
- Needing to be in control.
- Feeling helpless.
- Wanting to grasp or keep hold of what you have.
- Wanting to push away or eliminate your rival.

Expressions and Actions of Jealousy

- Violent behavior or threats of violence toward the person threatening to take something away.
- Attempting to control the freedom of the person you are afraid of losing.
- Verbal accusations of disloyalty or unfaithfulness.
- Spying on the person.
- Interrogating the person; demanding accounting of time or activities.
- Collecting evidence of wrongdoings.
- Clinging; enhanced dependency.
- Increased or excessive demonstrations of love.
- Other: _____

Aftereffects of Jealousy

- Narrowing of attention.
- Seeing the worst in others.
- Being mistrustful across the board.
- Being hypervigilant to threats to your relationships.
- Becoming isolated or withdrawn.
- Other: _____

(*continued on next page*)

LOVE WORDS

love	attraction	enchantment	limerence	sympathy
adoration	caring	fondness	longing	tenderness
affection	charmed	infatuation	lust	warmth
arousal	compassion	kindness	passion	
	desire	liking	sentimentality	

Prompting Events for Feeling Love

- A person:
  - Offers or gives you something you want, need, or desire.
  - Does things you want or need.
  - Does things you particularly value or admire.
- Feeling physically attracted to someone.
- Being with someone you have fun with.

- You spend a lot of time with a person.
- You share a special experience with a person.
- You have exceptionally good communication with a person.
- Other: _____

Interpretations of Events That Prompt Feelings of Love

- Believing that a person loves, needs, or appreciates you.
- Thinking that a person is physically attractive.
- Judging a person's personality as wonderful, pleasing, or attractive.
- Believing that a person can be counted on, or will always be there for you.
- Other: _____

Biological Changes and Experiences of Love

- When you are with or thinking about someone:
  - Feeling excited and full of energy.
  - Fast heartbeat.
  - Feeling self-confident.
  - Feeling invulnerable.
  - Feeling happy, joyful, or exuberant.
  - Feeling warm, trusting, and secure.
  - Feeling relaxed and calm.

- Wanting the best for a person.
- Wanting to give things to a person.
- Wanting to see and spend time with a person.
- Wanting to spend your life with a person.
- Wanting physical closeness or sex.
- Wanting emotional closeness.

Expressions and Actions of Love

- Saying "I love you."
- Expressing positive feelings to a person.
- Eye contact, mutual gaze.
- Touching, petting, hugging, holding, cuddling.
- Sexual activity.

- Smiling.
- Sharing time and experiences with someone.
- Doing things that the other person wants or needs.
- Other: _____

Aftereffects of Love

- Only seeing a person's positive side.
- Feeling forgetful or distracted; daydreaming.
- Feeling openness and trust.
- Feeling "alive," capable.
- Remembering other people you have loved.

- Remembering other people who have loved you.
- Remembering other positive events.
- Believing in yourself; believing you are wonderful, capable, competent.
- Other: _____

(*continued on next page*)

SADNESS WORDS

sadness	disappointment	pity	crushed	disconnected	depression
despair	homesickness	anguish	displeasure	suffering	glumness
grief	neglect	dismay	insecurity	dejection	melancholy
misery	alienation	hurt	sorrow	gloom	alone
agony	discontentment	rejection	defeat	loneliness	woe
			distraught	unhappiness	

Prompting Events for Feeling Sadness

- Losing something or someone irretrievably.
- The death of someone you love.
- Things not being what you expected or wanted.
- Things being worse than you expected.
- Being separated from someone you care for.
- Getting what you don't want.
- Not getting what you have worked for.
- Not getting what you believe you need in life.
- Being rejected, disapproved of, or excluded.
- Discovering that you are powerless or helpless.
- Being with someone else who is sad or in pain.
- Reading or hearing about other people's problems or troubles in the world.
- Being alone, or feeling isolated or like an outsider.
- Thinking about everything you have not gotten.
- Thinking about your losses.
- Thinking about missing someone.
- Other: _____

Interpretations of Events That Prompt Feelings of Sadness

- Believing that a separation from someone will last for a long time or will never end.
- Believing that you will not get what you want or need in your life.
- Seeing things or your life as hopeless.
- Believing that you are worthless or not valuable.
- Other: _____

Biological Changes and Experiences of Sadness

- Feeling tired, run down, or low in energy.
- Feeling lethargic, listless; wanting to stay in bed all day.
- Feeling as if nothing is pleasurable any more.
- Pain or hollowness in your chest or gut.
- Feeling empty.
- Feeling as if you can't stop crying, or if you ever start crying you will never be able to stop.
- Difficulty swallowing.
- Breathlessness.
- Dizziness.
- Other: _____

Expressions and Actions of Sadness

- Avoiding things.
- Acting helpless; staying in bed; being inactive.
- Moping, brooding, or acting moody.
- Making slow, shuffling movements.
- Withdrawing from social contact.
- Avoiding activities that used to bring pleasure.
- Giving up and no longer trying to improve.
- Saying sad things.
- Talking little or not at all.
- Using a quiet, slow, or monotonous voice.
- Eyes drooping.
- Frowning, not smiling.
- Posture slumping.
- Sobbing, crying, whimpering.
- Other: _____

Aftereffects of Sadness

- Not being able to remember happy things.
- Feeling irritable, touchy, or grouchy.
- Yearning and searching for the thing lost.
- Having a negative outlook.
- Blaming or criticizing yourself.
- Ruminating about sad events in the past.
- Insomnia.
- Appetite disturbance, indigestion.
- Other: _____

(*continued on next page*)

SHAME WORDS

shame	culpability	embarrassment	mortification	shyness
contrition	discomposure	humiliation	self-conscious	

Prompting Events for Feeling Shame

- Being rejected by people you care about.
- Having others find out that you have done something wrong.
- Doing (or feeling or thinking) something that people you admire believe is wrong or immoral.
- Comparing some aspect of yourself or your behavior to a standard and feeling as if you do not live up to that standard.
- Being betrayed by a person you love.
- Being laughed at/made fun of.
- Being criticized in public/in front of someone else; remembering public criticism.
- Others attacking your integrity.

- Being reminded of something wrong, immoral, or "shameful" you did in the past.
- Being rejected or criticized for something you expected praise for.
- Having emotions/experiences that have been invalidated.
- Exposure of a very private aspect of yourself or your life.
- Exposure of a physical characteristic you dislike.
- Failing at something you feel you are (or should be) competent to do.
- Other: _____

Interpretations of Events That Prompt Feelings of Shame

- Believing that others will reject you (or have rejected you).
- Judging yourself to be inferior, not "good enough," not as good as others; self-invalidation.
- Comparing yourself to others and thinking that you are a "loser."
- Believing yourself unlovable.
- Thinking that you are bad, immoral, or wrong.
- Thinking that you are defective.

- Thinking that you are a bad person or a failure.
- Believing your body (or a body part) is too big, too small, or ugly.
- Thinking that you have not lived up to others' expectations of you.
- Thinking that your behavior, thoughts, or feelings are silly or stupid.
- Other: _____

Biological Changes and Experiences of Shame

- Pain in the pit of the stomach.
- Sense of dread.
- Wanting to shrink down and/or disappear.

- Wanting to hide or cover your face and body.
- Other: _____

Expressions and Actions of Shame

- Hiding behavior or a characteristic from other people.
- Avoiding the person you have harmed.
- Avoiding persons who have criticized you.
- Avoiding yourself—distracting, ignoring.
- Withdrawing; covering the face.
- Bowing your head, groveling.

- Appeasing; saying you are sorry over and over and over.
- Looking down and away from others.
- Sinking back; slumped and rigid posture.
- Halting speech; lowered volume while talking.
- Other: _____

Aftereffects of Shame

- Avoiding thinking about your transgression; shutting down; blocking all emotions.
- Engaging in distracting, impulsive behaviors to divert your mind or attention.
- High amount of "self-focus"; preoccupation with yourself.
- Depersonalization, dissociative experiences,

numbness, or shock.
- Attacking or blaming others.
- Conflicts with other people.
- Isolation, feeling alienated.
- Impairment in problem-solving ability.
- Other: _____

(*continued on next page*)

GUILT WORDS

guilt	culpability	remorse	apologetic	regret	sorry

Prompting Events for Feeling Guilt

- Doing or thinking something you believe is wrong.
- Doing or thinking something that violates your personal values.
- Not doing something you said that you would do.
- Committing a transgression against another person or something you value.

- Causing harm/damage to another person or object.
- Causing harm/damage to yourself.
- Being reminded of something wrong you did in the past.
- Other: _____

Interpretations of Events That Prompt Feelings of Guilt

- Thinking that your actions are to blame for something.
- Thinking that you behaved badly.

- Thinking, "If only I had done something differently . . . "
- Other: _____

Biological Changes and Experiences of Guilt

- Hot, red face.
- Jitteriness, nervousness.

- Suffocating.
- Other: _____

Expressions and Actions of Guilt

- Trying to repair the harm, make amends for the wrongdoing, fix the damage, change the outcome.
- Asking for forgiveness, apologizing, confessing.
- Giving gifts/making sacrifices to try to make up for the transgression.
- Bowing your head; kneeling before the person.

Aftereffects of Guilt

- Making resolutions to change.
- Making changes in behavior.
- Joining self-help programs.
- Other: _____

Other Important Emotion Words

- Weariness, dissatisfaction, disinclination.
- Distress.
- Shyness, fragility, reserve, bashfulness, coyness, reticence.
- Cautiousness, reluctance, suspiciousness, caginess, wariness.
- Surprise, amazement, astonishment, awe, startle, wonder.
- Boldness, bravery, courage, determination.
- Powerfulness, a sense of competence, capability, mastery.
- Dubiousness, skepticism, doubtfulness.
- Apathy, boredom, dullness, ennui, fidgetiness, impatience, indifference, listlessness.

....

Handouts for Changing
Emotional Responses

....

Overview:
Changing Emotional Responses

CHECK THE FACTS

Check out whether your emotional reactions **fit the facts**
of the situation.

Changing your beliefs and assumptions to fit the facts can help
you change your emotional reactions to situations.

OPPOSITE ACTION

When your emotions do not fit the facts,
or when acting on your emotions is not effective,
acting opposite (all the way)
will change your emotional reactions.

PROBLEM SOLVING

When the facts themselves are the problem,
solving the problem
will reduce the frequency of negative emotions.

Check the Facts

FACTS

Many emotions and actions are set off by our thoughts and interpretations of events, not by the events themselves.

Event → Thoughts → Emotions

Our emotions can also have a big effect on our thoughts about events.

Event → Emotion → Thoughts

Examining our thoughts and *checking the facts* can help us change our emotions.

HOW TO CHECK THE FACTS

1. **Ask: What is the emotion I want to change?**
   (See Emotion Regulation Handout 6: Ways of Describing Emotions.)

2. **Ask: What is the event prompting my emotion?**
   Describe the facts that you observed through your senses.
   Challenge judgments, absolutes, and black-and-white descriptions.
   (See Mindfulness Handout 4: Taking Hold of Your Mind: "What" Skills.)

3. **Ask: What are my interpretations, thoughts, and assumptions about the event?**
   Think of other possible interpretations.
   Practice looking at all sides of a situation and all points of view.
   Test your interpretations and assumptions to see if they fit the facts.

4. **Ask: Am I assuming a threat?**
   Label the threat.
   Assess the probability that the threatening event will really occur.
   Think of as many other possible outcomes as you can.

5. **Ask: What's the catastrophe?**
   Imagine the catastrophe really occurring.
   Imagine coping well with a catastrophe (through problem solving, coping ahead, or radical acceptance).

6. **Ask: Does my emotion and/or its intensity fit the actual facts?**
   Check out facts that fit each emotion.
   Ask Wise Mind.
   (See Emotion Regulation Handout 11: Figuring Out Opposite Actions, and Emotion Regulation Handout 13: Reviewing Problem Solving and Opposite Action.)

Examples of Emotions That Fit the Facts

Fear	1. There is a threat to your life or that of someone you care about. 2. There is a threat to your health or that of someone you care about. 3. There is a threat to your well-being or that of someone you care about. 4. Other: _____
Anger	1. An important goal is blocked or a desired activity is interrupted or prevented. 2. You or someone you care about is attacked or hurt by others. 3. You or someone you care about is insulted or threatened by others. 4. The integrity or status of your social group is offended or threatened. 5. Other: _____
Disgust	1. Something you are in contact with could poison or contaminate you. 2. Somebody whom you deeply dislike is touching you or someone you care about. 3. You are around a person or group whose behavior or thinking could seriously damage or harmfully influence you or the group you are part of. 4. Other: _____
Envy	1. Another person or group gets or has things you don't have that you want or need. 2. Other: _____
Jealousy	1. A very important and desired relationship or object in your life is in danger of being damaged or lost. 2. Someone is threatening to take a valued relationship or object away from you. 3. Other: _____
Love	1. Loving a person, animal, or object enhances quality of life for you or for those you care about. 2. Loving a person, animal, or object increases your chances of attaining your own personal goals. 3. Other: _____
Sadness	1. You have lost something or someone permanently. 2. Things are not the way you wanted or expected and hoped them to be. 3. Other: _____
Shame	1. You will be rejected by a person or group you care about if characteristics of yourself or of your behavior are made public. 2. Other: _____
Guilt	1. Your own behavior violates your own values or moral code. 2. Other: _____

Intensity and duration of an emotion are justified by:

1. How likely it is that the expected outcomes will occur.
2. How great and/or important the outcomes are.
3. How effective the emotion is in your life now.

Opposite Action and Problem Solving:
Deciding Which to Use

Opposite action = Acting opposite to an emotion's action urge

Problem solving = Avoiding or changing (solving) a problem event

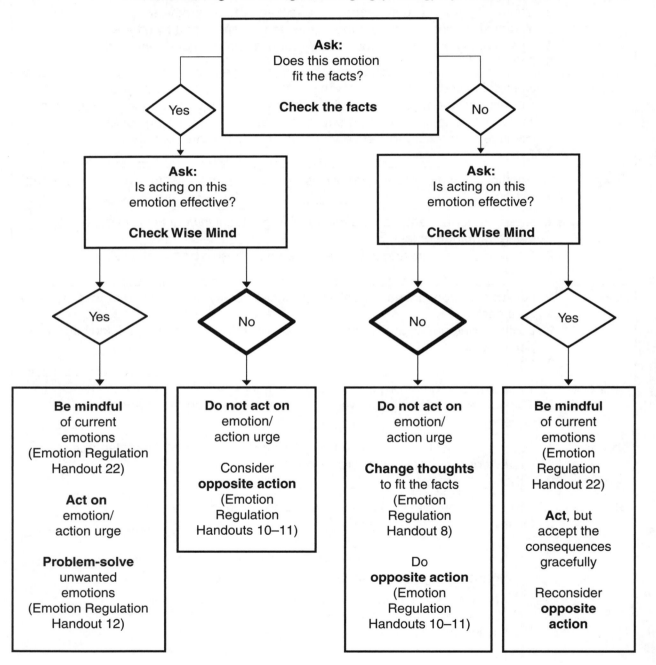

Ask:
Does this emotion
fit the facts?

Check the facts

Yes

No

Ask:
Is acting on this
emotion effective?

Check Wise Mind

Ask:
Is acting on this
emotion effective?

Check Wise Mind

Yes

No

No

Yes

Be mindful
of current
emotions
(Emotion Regulation
Handout 22)

Act on
emotion/
action urge

Problem-solve
unwanted
emotions
(Emotion Regulation
Handout 12)

Do not act on
emotion/
action urge

Consider
opposite action
(Emotion
Regulation
Handouts 10–11)

Do not act on
emotion/
action urge

Change thoughts
to fit the facts
(Emotion
Regulation
Handout 8)

Do
opposite action
(Emotion
Regulation
Handouts 10–11)

Be mindful
of current
emotions
(Emotion
Regulation
Handout 22)

Act, but
accept the
consequences
gracefully

Reconsider
**opposite
action**

Opposite Action

Use opposite action when your emotions do NOT fit the facts
or when acting on your emotions is NOT effective.

EVERY EMOTION HAS AN ACTION URGE.

CHANGE THE EMOTION BY <u>ACTING OPPOSITE</u> TO ITS ACTION URGE.

Consider these examples:

EMOTION	ACTION URGE	OPPOSITE ACTION
Fear	Run away/avoid	Approach/don't avoid
Anger	Attack	Gently avoid/be a little nice
Sadness	Withdraw/isolate	Get active
Shame	Hide/avoid	Tell the secret to people who will accept it

---

HOW TO DO OPPOSITE ACTION, STEP BY STEP

Step 1. **IDENTIFY AND NAME THE EMOTION** you want to change.

Step 2. **CHECK THE FACTS** to see if your emotion is justified by the facts.
Check also whether the intensity and duration of the emotion fit the facts.
(*Example: "Irritation" fits the facts when your car is cut in front of; "road rage" does not.*)
An emotion is justified when your emotion fits the facts.

Step 3. **IDENTIFY AND DESCRIBE YOUR ACTION URGES.**

Step 4. **ASK WISE MIND:** Is expression or acting on this emotion effective in this situation?

If your emotion does not fit the facts or if acting on your emotion is not effective:

Step 5. **IDENTIFY OPPOSITE ACTIONS** to your action urges.

Step 6. **ACT OPPOSITE <u>ALL THE WAY</u>** to your action urges.

Step 7. **REPEAT ACTING OPPOSITE** to your action urges until your emotion changes.

Figuring Out Opposite Actions

FEAR

Fear FITS THE FACTS of a situation whenever there is a THREAT to:

A. Your life or that of someone you care about.

B. Your health or that of someone you care about.

C. Your well-being or that of someone you care about.

D. Other example: _____

Follow these suggestions when your fear is NOT JUSTIFIED by the facts or NOT EFFECTIVE:

OPPOSITE ACTIONS for Fear

Do the OPPOSITE of your fearful action urges. For example:

1. Do what you are afraid of doing . . . OVER AND OVER.

2. APPROACH events, places, tasks, activities, and people you are afraid of.

3. Do things to give yourself a sense of CONTROL and MASTERY over your fears.

ALL-THE-WAY OPPOSITE ACTIONS for Fear

4. Keep your EYES AND EARS OPEN and focused on the feared event.

Look around slowly; explore.

5. Take in the information from the situation (i.e., notice that you are safe).

6. Change POSTURE AND KEEP A CONFIDENT VOICE TONE.

Keep your head and eyes up, and your shoulders back but relaxed.
Adopt an assertive body posture (e.g., knees apart, hands on hips, heels a bit out).

7. Change your BODY CHEMISTRY.

For example, do paced breathing by breathing in deeply and breathing out slowly.

(continued on next page)

ANGER

Anger FITS THE FACTS of a situation whenever:

A. An important goal is blocked or a desired activity is interrupted or prevented.

B. You or someone you care about is attacked or hurt by others.

C. You or someone you care about is insulted or threatened by others.

D. The integrity or status of your social group is offended or threatened.

E. Other example: _____

Follow these suggestions when your anger is NOT JUSTIFIED by the facts or is NOT EFFECTIVE:

OPPOSITE ACTIONS for Anger

Do the OPPOSITE of your angry action urges. For example:

1. GENTLY AVOID the person you are angry with (rather than attacking).

2. TAKE A TIME OUT, and breathe in and out deeply and slowly.

3. BE KIND (rather than mean or insulting).

ALL-THE-WAY OPPOSITE ACTIONS for Anger

4. IMAGINE UNDERSTANDING and empathy for the other person.

Step into the other person's shoes. Try to see the situation from the other person's point of view.
Imagine really good reasons for what has happened.

5. CHANGE YOUR POSTURE.

Unclench hands, with palms up and fingers relaxed (WILLING HANDS).
Relax chest and stomach muscles.
Unclench teeth.
Relax facial muscles. Half-smile.

6. CHANGE YOUR BODY CHEMISTRY.

For example, do paced breathing by breathing in deeply and breathing out slowly.
Or, run or engage in another physically energetic, nonviolent activity.

(*continued on next page*)

DISGUST

Disgust FITS THE FACTS of a situation whenever:

A. Something you are in contact with could poison or contaminate you.

B. Somebody whom you deeply dislike is touching you or someone you care about.

C. You are around a person or group whose behavior or thinking could seriously damage or harmfully influence you or the group you are part of.

D. Other example: _____

Follow these suggestions when your disgust is NOT JUSTIFIED by the facts or is NOT EFFECTIVE:

OPPOSITE ACTIONS for Disgust

Do the OPPOSITE of your disgusted action urges. For example:

1. MOVE CLOSE. Eat, drink, stand near, or embrace what you found disgusting.

2. Be KIND to those you feel contempt for; step into the other person's shoes.

ALL-THE-WAY OPPOSITE ACTIONS for Disgust

3. IMAGINE UNDERSTANDING and empathy for the person you feel disgust or contempt for.

Try to see the situation from the other person's point of view.
Imagine really good reasons for how the other person is behaving or looking.

4. TAKE IN what feels repulsive.

Be sensual (inhaling, looking at, touching, listening, tasting).

5. CHANGE YOUR POSTURE.

Unclench hands with palms up and fingers relaxed (willing hands).
Relax chest and stomach muscles.
Unclench teeth.
Relax facial muscles.
Half-smile.

6. CHANGE YOUR BODY CHEMISTRY.

For example, do paced breathing by breathing in deeply and breathing out slowly.

(*continued on next page*)

ENVY

Envy FITS THE FACTS of a situation whenever:

A. Another person or group has what you want or need but don't have.

B. Other example: _____

Follow these suggestions when your envy is NOT JUSTIFIED by the facts or is NOT EFFECTIVE:

OPPOSITE ACTIONS for Envy

Do the OPPOSITE of your envious action urges. For example:

1. INHIBIT DESTROYING what the other person has.

2. COUNT YOUR BLESSINGS. Make a list of the things you are thankful for.

ALL-THE-WAY OPPOSITE ACTIONS for Envy

3. COUNT ALL your blessings.

   Avoid discounting some blessings.
   Avoid exaggerating your deprivations.

4. Stop EXAGGERATING others' net worth or value; check the facts.

5. CHANGE YOUR POSTURE.

   Unclench hands with palms up and fingers relaxed (WILLING HANDS).
   Relax chest and stomach muscles.
   Unclench teeth.
   Relax facial muscles.
   Half-smile.

6. CHANGE YOUR BODY CHEMISTRY.

   For example, do paced breathing by breathing in deeply and breathing out slowly.

(continued on next page)

JEALOUSY

Jealousy FITS THE FACTS of a situation whenever:

A. Someone is threatening to take a very important and desired relationship or object away from you.

B. An important and desired relationship is in danger of being damaged or lost.

C. Other example: _____

Follow these suggestions when your jealousy is NOT JUSTIFIED by the facts or is NOT EFFECTIVE:

OPPOSITE ACTIONS for Jealousy

Do the OPPOSITE of your jealous action urges. For example:

1. LET GO of controlling others' actions.

2. SHARE the things and people you have in your life.

ALL-THE-WAY OPPOSITE ACTIONS for Jealousy

3. STOP SPYING or snooping.

Suppress probing questions ("Where were you? Who were you with?").
Fire your "private detective."

4. NO AVOIDING. Listen to all the details. Focus on sensations.

Keep your eyes open; look around.
Take in all the information about the situation.

5. CHANGE YOUR POSTURE.

Unclench hands with palms up and fingers relaxed (WILLING HANDS).
Relax chest and stomach muscles.
Unclench teeth.
Relax facial muscles.
Half-smile.

6. CHANGE YOUR BODY CHEMISTRY.

For example, do paced breathing by breathing in deeply and breathing out slowly.

(*continued on next page*)

LOVE

Love (other than universal love for all) FITS THE FACTS of a situation whenever:

A. Loving a person, animal, or object enhances quality of life for you or for those you care about.

B. Loving a person, animal, or object increases your chances of attaining your own personal goals.

C. Other example: _____

Follow these suggestions when your love is NOT JUSTIFIED by the facts or is NOT EFFECTIVE:

OPPOSITE ACTIONS for Love

Do the OPPOSITE of your loving action urges. For example:

1. AVOID the person, animal, or object you love.

2. DISTRACT yourself from thoughts of the person, animal, or object.

3. REMIND yourself of why love is not justified (rehearse the "cons" of loving) when loving thoughts do arise.

ALL-THE-WAY OPPOSITE ACTIONS for Love

4. AVOID CONTACT with everything that reminds you of a person you love: pictures, letters/messages/e-mails, belongings, mementos, places you were together, places you planned to or wanted to go together, places where you know the person has been or will be. No following, waiting for, or looking for the person.

5. STOP EXPRESSING LOVE for the person, even to friends. Be unfriendly toward the person (e.g., "unfriend" the person on Facebook, Twitter, etc.).

6. ADJUST YOUR POSTURE AND EXPRESSIONS if you are around the person you love.

No leaning toward him or her.
No getting close enough to touch.
No sighing/gazing at the person.

(*continued on next page*)

SADNESS

Sadness FITS THE FACTS of a situation whenever:

A. You have lost something or someone permanently.

B. Things are not the way you want or expected and hoped them to be.

C. Other example: _____

Follow these suggestions when sadness is NOT JUSTIFIED by the facts or is NOT EFFECTIVE:

OPPOSITE ACTIONS for Sadness

Do the OPPOSITE of your sad action (or inaction) urges. For example:

1. Get ACTIVE; approach.

2. AVOID AVOIDING.

3. BUILD MASTERY: Do things that make you feel competent and self-confident.
   (See Emotion Regulation Handout 19: Build Mastery and Cope Ahead.)

4. Increase PLEASANT EVENTS.

ALL-THE-WAY OPPOSITE ACTIONS for Sadness

5. Pay attention to the PRESENT MOMENT!

   Be mindful of your environment—each detail as it unfolds.
   Experience new or positive activities you are engaging in.

6. CHANGE YOUR POSTURE (adopt a "bright" body posture, with head up, eyes open, and shoulders back).

   Keep an upbeat voice tone.

7. CHANGE YOUR BODY CHEMISTRY.

   For example, increase physical movement (run, jog, walk, or do other active exercise).

(continued on next page)

SHAME

Shame FITS THE FACTS of a situation whenever:

A. You will be rejected by a person or group you care about if your personal characteristics or behavior are made public.

B. Other example: _____

Follow these suggestions when *both* shame and guilt
are NOT JUSTIFIED by the facts or are NOT EFFECTIVE:

OPPOSITE ACTIONS for Shame

Do the OPPOSITE of your action urges. For example:

1. MAKE PUBLIC your personal characteristics or your behavior (with people who won't reject you).

2. REPEAT the behavior that sets off shame over and over (without hiding the behavior from those who won't reject you).

ALL-THE-WAY OPPOSITE ACTIONS for Shame

3. NO APOLOGIZING or trying to make up for a perceived transgression.

4. TAKE IN all the information from the situation.

5. CHANGE YOUR BODY POSTURE. Look innocent and proud. Lift your head; "puff up" your chest; maintain eye contact. Keep your voice tone steady and clear.

Follow these suggestions when shame is NOT JUSTIFIED by the facts or is NOT EFFECTIVE, but *GUILT IS JUSTIFIED* (your behavior does violate your own moral values):

OPPOSITE ACTIONS for Shame

Do the OPPOSITE of your action urges. For example:

1. MAKE PUBLIC your behavior (with people who won't reject you).

2. APOLOGIZE for your behavior.

3. REPAIR the transgressions, or work to prevent or repair similar harm for others.

4. COMMIT to avoiding that mistake in the future.

5. ACCEPT the consequences gracefully.

ALL-THE-WAY OPPOSITE ACTIONS for Shame

6. FORGIVE yourself. Acknowledge the causes of your behavior.

7. LET IT GO.

(*continued on next page*)

GUILT

Guilt FITS THE FACTS of a situation whenever:

A. Your behavior violates your own values or moral code.

B. Other example: _____

Follow these suggestions when *both* guilt and shame
are NOT JUSTIFIED by the facts or are NOT EFFECTIVE:

OPPOSITE ACTIONS for Guilt

Do the OPPOSITE of your action urges. For example:

1. MAKE PUBLIC your personal characteristics or your behavior (with people who won't reject you).

2. REPEAT the behavior that sets off guilt over and over (without hiding the behavior from those who won't reject you).

ALL-THE-WAY OPPOSITE ACTIONS for Guilt

3. NO APOLOGIZING or trying to make up for a perceived transgression.

4. TAKE IN all the information from the situation.

5. CHANGE YOUR BODY POSTURE. Look innocent and proud. Lift your head; "puff up" your chest; maintain eye contact. Keep your voice tone steady and clear.

Follow these suggestions when guilt is NOT JUSTIFIED by the facts or is NOT EFFECTIVE
but SHAME IS JUSTIFIED (you will be rejected by people you care about if found out):

OPPOSITE ACTIONS for Guilt

1. HIDE your behavior (if you want to stay in the group).

2. USE INTERPERSONAL SKILLS (if you want to stay in the group).

3. WORK TO CHANGE the person's or group's values.

4. JOIN A NEW GROUP that fits your values (and will not reject you).

5. REPEAT the behavior that sets off guilt over and over with your new group.

ALL-THE-WAY OPPOSITE ACTIONS for Guilt

6. VALIDATE YOURSELF.

Problem Solving

Step 1. FIGURE OUT and DESCRIBE the problem situation.

Step 2. CHECK THE FACTS (*all* the facts) to be sure you have the right problem situation!

If your facts are correct and the situation is the problem, ***continue with* STEP 3.**

If your facts are not correct, ***go back and repeat* STEP 1.**

Step 3. IDENTIFY YOUR GOAL in solving the problem.
- Identify what needs to happen or change for you to feel OK.
- Keep it simple, and choose something that can actually happen.

Step 4. BRAINSTORM lots of solutions.
- Think of as many solutions as you can. Ask for suggestions from people you trust.
- Do not be critical of any ideas at first. (Wait for Step 5 to evaluate ideas.)

Step 5. CHOOSE a solution that fits the goal and is likely to work.
- If you are unsure, choose two solutions that look good.
- Do PROS and CONS to compare the solutions.
- Choose the best to try first.

Step 6. Put the solution into ACTION.
- ACT! Try out the solution.
- Take the first step, and then the second . . .

Step 7. EVALUATE the results of using the solution.

It worked? **YEA!!!**   *It didn't work?* ***Go back to* STEP 5** and choose a new solution to try.

Reviewing Opposite Action and Problem Solving

	Justifying Events	Act Opposite to Emotion Urge (for Unjustified Emotion)	Act on Emotion Urge, Problem-Solve, or Avoid (for Justified Emotion)
Fear	**A.** Your life is in danger. **B.** Your health is in danger. **C.** Your well-being is in danger.	**1.** Do what you are afraid of doing . . . over and over. **2.** Approach what you are afraid of. **3.** Do what gives you a sense of control and mastery.	**1.** Freeze/run if danger is near. **2.** Remove the threatening event. **3.** Do what gives you a sense of control and mastery of the fearful event. **4.** Avoid the threatening event.
Anger	**A.** An important goal is blocked or a desired activity is interrupted or prevented. **B.** You or someone you care about is attacked or hurt (physically or emotionally) by others. **C.** You or someone you care about is insulted, offended, or threatened by others.	**1.** Gently avoid. **2.** Take a time out. **3.** Do something kind. **4.** Imagine understanding: Step into the other person's shoes. **5.** Imagine really good reasons for what happened.	**1.** Fight back when being attacked, if you have nothing to lose by fighting. **2.** Overcome obstacles to goals. **3.** Work to stop further attacks, insults, and threats. **4.** Avoid or walk out on people who are threatening.
Disgust	**A.** Something you are in contact with could poison or contaminate you. **B.** You are close to a person or group whose actions or thinking could seriously damage or harm you or the group you are part of.	**1.** Move close. Embrace. **2.** Be kind; step into the other person's shoes. **3.** Take in what feels repulsive. **4.** See the situation from the other person's point of view.	**1.** Remove/clean up revolting things. **2.** Influence others to stop harmful actions/stop things that contaminate your community. **3.** Avoid or push away harmful people or things. **4.** Imagine understanding a person who has done disgusting things.

(*continued on next page*)

	Justifying Events	Act Opposite to Emotion Urge (for Unjustified Emotion)	Act on Emotion Urge, Problem-Solve, or Avoid (for Justified Emotion)
Envy	**A.** Another person or group gets or has things you don't have that you want or need.	**1.** Inhibit destroying other people's things. **2.** Count your blessings. **3.** Imagine how it all makes sense. **4.** Stop exaggerating others' worth or value.	**1.** Improve yourself and your life. **2.** Get others to be fair. **3.** Devalue what others have that you don't have. **4.** Put on rose-colored glasses. **5.** Avoid people who have more than you.
Jealousy	**A.** An important and desired relationship or object is in danger of being damaged or lost. **B.** Someone is threatening to take away an important and desired relationship or object.	**1.** Let go of trying to control others. **2.** Share what you have with others. **3.** Stop spying and snooping. **4.** No avoiding; take in all the information.	**1.** Protect what you have. **2.** Work at being more desirable to the person(s) you want to be in a relationship with (i.e., fight for relationships). **3.** Leave the relationship.
Love	**A.** Loving a valued/admired person, animal, or object enhances the quality of life for you or those you care about. **B.** Loving the person, animal, or object increases your chances of attaining your own personal goals.	**1.** Avoid the person, animal, or object you love altogether. **2.** Distract yourself from thoughts of the beloved. **3.** Avoid contact with all reminders of the beloved. **4.** Remind yourself of why love is not justified.	**1.** Be with the person, animal, or thing that you love. **2.** Touch, hold, etc., the beloved. **3.** Avoid separations when possible. **4.** If the beloved is lost, fight to find or get the beloved back (if it may be possible).
Sadness	**A.** You have lost something or someone permanently. **B.** Things are not the way you expected or wanted or hoped for.	**1.** Activate your behavior. **2.** Avoid avoiding. **3.** Build mastery: Do things that make you feel competent and self-confident. **4.** Increase pleasant events. **5.** Pay attention to pleasant events.	**1.** Grieve; have a memorial service; visit the cemetery (but don't build a house at the cemetery). **2.** Retrieve/replace what is lost. **3.** Plan how to rebuild a life worth living without the beloved or expected outcomes in your life. **4.** Accumulate positives. **5.** Build mastery: Do things that make you feel competent and self-confident. **6.** Communicate need for help. **7.** Accept help offered. **8.** Put on rose-colored glasses.

(*continued on next page*)

	Justifying Events	Act Opposite to Emotion Urge (for Unjustified Emotion)	Act on Emotion Urge, Problem-Solve, or Avoid (for Justified Emotion)
Shame	A. You will be rejected by a very important person or group if characteristics of yourself or of your behavior are made public.	1. Make public your personal characteristics or behavior (with people who won't reject you). 2. Repeat the behavior without hiding from people who won't reject you. 3. Or, if *your* moral code is violated, apologize and repair; forgive yourself; and let it go.	1. Hide what will get you rejected. 2. Appease those offended. 3. Change your behavior or personal characteristics to fit in. 4. Avoid groups who disapprove of you. 5. Find a new group that fits your values or that likes your personal characteristics. 6. Work to change society's or a person's values.
Guilt	A. Your own behavior violates your own values or moral code.	1. Do what makes you feel guilty over and over and over. 2. Make public your behavior (with people who won't reject you). Or, if *you will be rejected by others:* 3. Hide your behavior. 4. Use interpersonal skills. 5. Work to change your group's values or join a new group.	1. Seek forgiveness. 2. Repair the harm; make things better (or, if not possible, work to prevent or repair similar harm for others). 3. Accept the consequences gracefully. 4. Commit to avoiding behaviors that violate your moral values in the future.

Handouts for Reducing Vulnerability to Emotion Mind

Overview:
Reducing Vulnerability to Emotion Mind—
Building a Life Worth Living

A way to remember these skills is to remember the term **ABC PLEASE.**

A

ACCUMULATE POSITIVE EMOTIONS

Short Term: Do pleasant things that are possible now.

Long Term: Make changes in your life so that positive events will happen more often in the future. Build a "life worth living."

B

BUILD MASTERY

Do things that make you feel competent and effective to combat helplessness and hopelessness.

C

COPE AHEAD OF TIME
WITH EMOTIONAL SITUATIONS

Rehearse a plan ahead of time so that you are prepared to cope skillfully with emotional situations.

PLEASE

TAKE CARE OF YOUR MIND
BY TAKING CARE OF YOUR BODY

Treat **P**hysica**L** illness, balance **E**ating,
avoid mood-**A**ltering substances, balance **S**leep,
and get **E**xercise.

Accumulating Positive Emotions: Short Term

Accumulate positive emotions in the short term by doing these things.

BUILD POSITIVE EXPERIENCES <u>NOW</u>

- INCREASE PLEASANT EVENTS that lead to positive emotions.
- Do ONE THING each day from the Pleasant Events List.
  (See Emotion Regulation Handout 16.)
- Practice opposite action; AVOID AVOIDING.
- BE MINDFUL of pleasant events (no multitasking).

BE MINDFUL OF POSITIVE EXPERIENCES

- FOCUS your attention on positive moments when they are happening. No multitasking.
- REFOCUS your attention when your mind wanders to the negative.
- PARTICIPATE and ENGAGE fully in each experience.

BE UNMINDFUL OF WORRIES

Such as . . .

- When the positive experience will end.
- Whether you deserve this positive experience.
- How much more might be expected of you now.

Pleasant Events List

1. ❑ Working on my car
2. ❑ Planning a career
3. ❑ Getting out of (paying down) debt
4. ❑ Collecting things (baseball cards, coins, stamps, rocks, shells, etc.)
5. ❑ Going on vacation
6. ❑ Thinking how it will be when I finish school
7. ❑ Recycling old items
8. ❑ Going on a date
9. ❑ Relaxing
10. ❑ Going to or watching a movie
11. ❑ Jogging, walking
12. ❑ Thinking, "I have done a full day's work"
13. ❑ Listening to music
14. ❑ Thinking about past parties
15. ❑ Buying household gadgets
16. ❑ Lying in the sun
17. ❑ Planning a career change
18. ❑ Laughing
19. ❑ Thinking about past trips
20. ❑ Listening to other people
21. ❑ Reading magazines or newspapers
22. ❑ Engaging in hobbies (stamp collecting, model building, etc.)
23. ❑ Spending an evening with good friends
24. ❑ Planning a day's activities
25. ❑ Meeting new people
26. ❑ Remembering beautiful scenery
27. ❑ Saving money
28. ❑ Going home from work
29. ❑ Eating
30. ❑ Practicing karate, judo, yoga
31. ❑ Thinking about retirement
32. ❑ Repairing things around the house
33. ❑ Working on machinery (cars, boats, etc.)
34. ❑ Remembering the words and deeds of loving people
35. ❑ Wearing shocking clothes

36. ❑ Having quiet evenings
37. ❑ Taking care of my plants
38. ❑ Buying, selling stock
39. ❑ Going swimming
40. ❑ Doodling
41. ❑ Exercising
42. ❑ Collecting old things
43. ❑ Going to a party
44. ❑ Thinking about buying things
45. ❑ Playing golf
46. ❑ Playing soccer
47. ❑ Flying kites
48. ❑ Having discussions with friends
49. ❑ Having family get-togethers
50. ❑ Riding a bike or motorbike
51. ❑ Running track
52. ❑ Going camping
53. ❑ Singing around the house
54. ❑ Arranging flowers
55. ❑ Practicing religion (going to church, group praying, etc.)
56. ❑ Organizing tools
57. ❑ Going to the beach
58. ❑ Thinking, "I'm an OK person"
59. ❑ Having a day with nothing to do
60. ❑ Going to class reunions
61. ❑ Going skating, skateboarding, rollerblading
62. ❑ Going sailing or motorboating
63. ❑ Traveling or going on vacations
64. ❑ Painting
65. ❑ Doing something spontaneously
66. ❑ Doing needlepoint, crewel, etc.
67. ❑ Sleeping
68. ❑ Driving
69. ❑ Entertaining, giving parties
70. ❑ Going to clubs (garden clubs, Parents without Partners, etc.)
71. ❑ Thinking about getting married
72. ❑ Going hunting

(**continued on next page**)

Note. For adults or adolescents. Adapted from Linehan, M. M., Sharp, E., & Ivanoff, A. M. (1980, November). *The Adult Pleasant Events Schedule.* Paper presented at the meeting of the Association for Advancement of Behavior Therapy, New York. Adapted by permission of the authors.

73. ❑ Singing with groups
74. ❑ Flirting
75. ❑ Playing musical instruments
76. ❑ Doing arts and crafts
77. ❑ Making a gift for someone
78. ❑ Buying/downloading music
79. ❑ Watching boxing, wrestling
80. ❑ Planning parties
81. ❑ Cooking
82. ❑ Going hiking
83. ❑ Writing (books, poems, articles)
84. ❑ Sewing
85. ❑ Buying clothes
86. ❑ Going out to dinner
87. ❑ Working
88. ❑ Discussing books; going to a book club
89. ❑ Sightseeing
90. ❑ Getting a manicure/pedicure or facial
91. ❑ Going to the beauty parlor
92. ❑ Early morning coffee and newspaper
93. ❑ Playing tennis
94. ❑ Kissing
95. ❑ Watching my children (play)
96. ❑ Thinking, "I have a lot more going for me than most people"
97. ❑ Going to plays and concerts
98. ❑ Daydreaming
99. ❑ Planning to go (back) to school
100. ❑ Thinking about sex
101. ❑ Going for a drive
102. ❑ Refinishing furniture
103. ❑ Watching TV
104. ❑ Making lists of tasks
105. ❑ Walking in the woods (or at the waterfront)
106. ❑ Buying gifts
107. ❑ Completing a task
108. ❑ Going to a spectator sport (auto racing, horse racing)
109. ❑ Teaching
110. ❑ Photography
111. ❑ Going fishing
112. ❑ Thinking about pleasant events
113. ❑ Staying on a diet
114. ❑ Playing with animals
115. ❑ Flying a plane
116. ❑ Reading fiction

117. ❑ Acting
118. ❑ Being alone
119. ❑ Writing diary entries or letters
120. ❑ Cleaning
121. ❑ Reading nonfiction
122. ❑ Taking children places
123. ❑ Dancing
124. ❑ Weightlifting
125. ❑ Going on a picnic
126. ❑ Thinking, "I did that pretty well," after doing something
127. ❑ Meditating, yoga
128. ❑ Having lunch with a friend
129. ❑ Going to the mountains
130. ❑ Playing hockey
131. ❑ Working with clay or pottery
132. ❑ Glass blowing
133. ❑ Going skiing
134. ❑ Dressing up
135. ❑ Reflecting on how I've improved
136. ❑ Buying small things for myself (perfume, golf balls, etc.)
137. ❑ Talking on the phone
138. ❑ Going to museums
139. ❑ Thinking religious thoughts
140. ❑ Lighting candles
141. ❑ White-water canoeing/rafting
142. ❑ Going bowling
143. ❑ Doing woodworking
144. ❑ Fantasizing about the future
145. ❑ Taking ballet/tap-dancing classes
146. ❑ Debating
147. ❑ Sitting in a sidewalk café
148. ❑ Having an aquarium
149. ❑ Participating in "living history" events
150. ❑ Knitting
151. ❑ Doing crossword puzzles
152. ❑ Shooting pool
153. ❑ Getting a massage
154. ❑ Saying, "I love you"
155. ❑ Playing catch, taking batting practice
156. ❑ Shooting baskets
157. ❑ Seeing and/or showing photos
158. ❑ Thinking about my good qualities
159. ❑ Solving riddles mentally
160. ❑ Having a political discussion
161. ❑ Buying books

(*continued on next page*)

162. ❑ Taking a sauna or a steam bath
163. ❑ Checking out garage sales
164. ❑ Thinking about having a family
165. ❑ Thinking about happy moments in my childhood
166. ❑ Splurging
167. ❑ Going horseback riding
168. ❑ Doing something new
169. ❑ Working on jigsaw puzzles
170. ❑ Playing cards
171. ❑ Thinking, "I'm a person who can cope"
172. ❑ Taking a nap
173. ❑ Figuring out my favorite scent
174. ❑ Making a card and giving it to someone I care about
175. ❑ Instant-messaging/texting someone
176. ❑ Playing a board game (e.g., Monopoly, Life, Clue, Sorry)
177. ❑ Putting on my favorite piece of clothing
178. ❑ Making a smoothie and drinking it slowly
179. ❑ Putting on makeup
180. ❑ Thinking about a friend's good qualities
181. ❑ Completing something I feel great about
182. ❑ Surprising someone with a favor
183. ❑ Surfing the Internet
184. ❑ Playing video games
185. ❑ E-mailing friends
186. ❑ Going walking or sledding in a snowfall
187. ❑ Getting a haircut
188. ❑ Installing new software
189. ❑ Buying a CD or music on iTunes
190. ❑ Watching sports on TV
191. ❑ Taking care of my pets
192. ❑ Doing volunteer service
193. ❑ Watching stand-up comedy on YouTube
194. ❑ Working in my garden
195. ❑ Participating in a public performance (e.g., a flash mob)
196. ❑ Blogging
197. ❑ Fighting for a cause
198. ❑ Conducting experiments

199. ❑ Expressing my love to someone
200. ❑ Going on field trips, nature walks, exploring (hiking away from known routes, spelunking)
201. ❑ Gathering natural objects (wild foods or fruit, driftwood)
202. ❑ Going downtown or to a shopping mall
203. ❑ Going to a fair, carnival, circus, zoo, or amusement park
204. ❑ Going to the library
205. ❑ Joining or forming a band
206. ❑ Learning to do something new
207. ❑ Listening to the sounds of nature
208. ❑ Looking at the moon or stars
209. ❑ Outdoor work (cutting or chopping wood, farm work)
210. ❑ Playing organized sports (baseball, softball, football, Frisbee, handball, paddleball, squash, soccer, tennis, volleyball, etc.)
211. ❑ Playing in the sand, a stream, the grass; kicking leaves, pebbles, etc.
212. ❑ Protesting social, political, or environmental conditions
213. ❑ Reading cartoons or comics
214. ❑ Reading sacred works
215. ❑ Rearranging or redecorating my room or the house
216. ❑ Selling or trading something
217. ❑ Snowmobiling or riding a dune buggy/ATV
218. ❑ Social networking
219. ❑ Soaking in the bathtub
220. ❑ Learning or speaking a foreign language
221. ❑ Talking on the phone
222. ❑ Composing or arranging songs or music
223. ❑ Thrift store shopping
224. ❑ Using computers
225. ❑ Visiting people who are sick, shut in, or in trouble

Other: _____

_____

_____

_____

Accumulating Positive Emotions: Long Term

A ccumulate positive emotions in the long term
to build a "life worth living."

That is, make changes in your life so that positive events will occur in the future.

Step 1. Avoid avoiding.

Start now to do what is needed to build the life you want. If you are not sure about what to do, follow the steps below.

Step 2. Identify values that are important to you.

ASK: What values are really important to me in my life?
Examples: Be productive; be part of a group; treat others well; be physically fit.

Step 3. Identify one value to work on now.

ASK: What is really important to me, right now, to work on in my life?
Example: Be productive.

Step 4. Identify a few goals related to this value.

ASK: What specific goals can I work on that will make this value part of my life?
Examples: Get a job where I can do something useful.
Be more active keeping up with important tasks at home.
Find a volunteer job that will use skills I already have.

Step 5. Choose one goal to work on now.

Do pros and cons, if necessary, to select a goal to work on now.
Example: Get a job where I can do something useful.

Step 6. Identify small action steps toward your goal.

ASK: What small steps can I take to get to my goal?
Examples: Visit places and look for job openings on the Internet in my area.
Submit applications for jobs at places I want to work.
Write résumé.
Check out benefits at places I might want to work.

Step 7. Take one action step now.
Example: Go on Internet and check for jobs in my area.

Values and Priorities List

In my own Wise Mind, I believe it is important to:

❑ A. Attend to relationships.

1. ❑ Repair old relationships.

2. ❑ Reach out for new relationships.

3. ❑ Work on current relationships.

4. ❑ End destructive relationships.

❑ Other: _____

❑ B. Be part of a group.

5. ❑ Have close and satisfying relationships with others.

6. ❑ Feel a sense of belonging.

7. ❑ Receive affection and love.

8. ❑ Be involved and intimate with others; have and keep close friends.

9. ❑ Have a family; stay close to and spend time with family members.

10. ❑ Have people to do things with.

❑ Other: _____

❑ C. Be powerful and able to influence others.

11. ❑ Have the authority to approve or disapprove of what people do, or to control how resources are used.

12. ❑ Be a leader.

13. ❑ Make a great deal of money.

14. ❑ Be respected by others.

15. ❑ Be seen by others as successful; become well known; obtain recognition and status.

16. ❑ Compete successfully with others.

17. ❑ Be popular and accepted.

❑ Other: _____

❑ D. Achieve things in life.

18. ❑ Achieve significant goals; be involved in undertakings I believe are significant.

19. ❑ Be productive.

20. ❑ Work toward goals; work hard.

21. ❑ Be ambitious.

❑ Other: _____

(*continued on next page*)

Adapted from Schwartz, S. H. (1992). Universals in the content and structure of values: Theory and empirical tests in 20 countries. In M. Zanna (Ed.), *Advances in experimental social psychology* (Vol. 25, pp. 1–65). New York: Academic Press. Copyright 1992 by Academic Press. Adapted by permission of Elsevier B.V.

❑ **E. Live a life of pleasure and satisfaction.**

    22. ❑ Have a good time.

    23. ❑ Seek fun and things that give pleasure.

    24. ❑ Have free time.

    25. ❑ Enjoy the work I do.

    ❑ Other: _____

❑ **F. Keep life full of exciting events, relationships, and things.**

    26. ❑ Try new and different things in life.

    27. ❑ Be daring and seek adventures.

    28. ❑ Have an exciting life.

    ❑ Other: _____

❑ **G. Behave respectfully.**

    29. ❑ Be humble and modest; do not draw attention to myself.

    30. ❑ Follow traditions and customs; behave properly.

    31. ❑ Do what I am told and follow rules.

    32. ❑ Treat others well.

    ❑ Other: _____

❑ **H. Be self-directed.**

    33. ❑ Follow my own path in life.

    34. ❑ Be innovative, think of new ideas, and be creative.

    35. ❑ Make my own decisions and be free.

    36. ❑ Be independent; take care of myself and those I am responsible for.

    37. ❑ Have freedom of thought and action; be able to act in terms of my own priorities.

    ❑ Other: _____

❑ **I. Be a spiritual person.**

    38. ❑ Make room in life for spirituality; live life according to spiritual principles.

    39. ❑ Practice a religion or faith.

    40. ❑ Grow in understanding of myself, my personal calling, and life's real purpose.

    41. ❑ Discern and do the will of God (or a higher power) and find lasting meaning in life.

    ❑ Other: _____

❑ **J. Be secure.**

    42. ❑ Live in secure and safe surroundings.

    43. ❑ Be physically healthy and fit.

    44. ❑ Have a steady income that meets my own and my family's basic needs.

    ❑ Other: _____

(*continued on next page*)

❑ **K. Recognize the universal good of all things.**

    45. ❑ Be fair, treat people equally, and provide equal opportunities.

    46. ❑ Understand different people; be open-minded.

    47. ❑ Care for nature and the environment.

        ❑ Other: _____

❑ **L. Contribute to the larger community.**

    48. ❑ Help people and those in need; care for others' well-being; improve society.

    49. ❑ Be loyal to friends and devoted to close people; be committed to a group that shares my beliefs, values, and ethical principles.

    50. ❑ Be committed to a cause or to a group that has a larger purpose beyond my own.

    51. ❑ Make sacrifices for others.

        ❑ Other: _____

❑ **M. Work at self-development.**

    52. ❑ Develop a personal philosophy of life.

    53. ❑ Learn and do challenging things that help me grow and mature as a human being.

        ❑ Other: _____

❑ **N. Have integrity.**

    54. ❑ Be honest, and acknowledge and stand up for my personal beliefs.

    55. ❑ Be a responsible person; keep my word to others.

    56. ❑ Be courageous in facing and living life.

    57. ❑ Be a person who pays debts to others and repairs damage I have caused.

    58. ❑ Be accepting of myself, others, and life as it is; live without resentment.

        ❑ Other: _____

❑ **O. Other:** _____

_____

_____

_____

Build Mastery and Cope Ahead

Build Mastery

1. Plan on doing at least one thing each day to build a sense of accomplishment.
   Example: _____

2. Plan for success, not failure.
   - Do something difficult, but possible.

3. Gradually increase the difficulty over time.
   - If the first task is too difficult, do something a little easier next time.

4. Look for a challenge.
   - If the task is too *easy*, try something a little harder next time.

Cope Ahead of Time with Difficult Situations

1. **Describe** the situation that is likely to prompt problem behavior.
   - Check the facts. Be specific in describing the situation.
   - Name the emotions and actions likely to interfere with using your skills.

2. **Decide** what coping or problem-solving skills you want to use in the situation.
   - Be specific. Write out in detail how you will cope with the situation and with your emotions and action urges.

3. **Imagine the situation** in your mind as vividly as possible.
   - Imagine yourself IN the situation NOW, not watching the situation.

4. **Rehearse in your mind coping effectively.**
   - Rehearse in your mind exactly what you can do to cope effectively.
   - Rehearse your actions, your thoughts, what you say, and how to say it.
   - Rehearse coping effectively with new problems that come up.
   - Rehearse coping effectively with your most feared catastrophe.

5. **Practice relaxation *after* rehearsing.**

Taking Care of Your Mind by Taking Care of Your Body

Remember these as **PLEASE** skills.

P

L

1. Treat PhysicaL Illness.

Take care of your body. See a doctor when necessary. Take prescribed medication.

E

2. Balance Eating.

Don't eat too much or too little. Eat regularly and mindfully throughout the day. Stay away from foods that make you feel overly emotional.

A

3. Avoid Mood-Altering Substances.

Stay off illicit drugs, and use alcohol in moderation (if at all).

S

4. Balance Sleep.

Try to get 7–9 hours of sleep a night, or at least the amount of sleep that helps you feel good. Keep to a consistent sleep schedule, especially if you are having difficulty sleeping.

E

5. Get Exercise.

Do some sort of exercise every day. Try to build up to 20 minutes of daily exercise.

Nightmare Protocol, Step by Step
When Nightmares Keep You from Sleeping

1. **Practice relaxation, pleasant imagery, and coping skills first, to be sure you are ready to work on changing your nightmares.**

   Do progressive relaxation, paced breathing, and/or Wise Mind exercises; listen to music or guided imagery; review the distress tolerance crisis survival skills.

2. **Choose a recurring nightmare you would like to work on.**

   This will be your target nightmare. Select a nightmare you can manage now. Put off trauma nightmares until you are ready to work with them—or, if you target a trauma nightmare, skip Step 3.

3. **Write down your target nightmare.**

   Include sensory descriptions (sights, smells, sounds, tastes, etc.). Also include any thoughts, feelings, and assumptions about yourself during the dream.

4. **Choose a changed outcome for the nightmare.**

   The change should occur BEFORE anything traumatic or bad happens to you or others in the nightmare. Essentially, you want to come up with a change that will prevent the bad outcome of the usual nightmare from occurring. Write an ending that will give you a sense of peace when you wake up.

   Note: Changes in the nightmare can be very unusual and out of the ordinary (e.g., you might become a person with superhuman powers who is able to escape to safety or fight off attackers). Changed outcomes can include changed thoughts, feelings, or assumptions about yourself.

5. **Write down the full nightmare with the changes.**

6. **REHEARSE and RELAX each night before going to sleep.**

   Rehearse the *changed* nightmare by visualizing the entire dream with the changes each night, *before* practicing relaxation techniques.

7. **REHEARSE and RELAX during the day.**

   Visualize the entire dream with the change, and practice relaxation as often as possible during the day.

Sleep Hygiene Protocol
When You Can't Sleep, What to Do Instead of Ruminating

TO INCREASE THE LIKELIHOOD OF RESTFULNESS/SLEEP:

1. **Develop and follow a consistent sleep schedule even on weekends.** Go to bed and get up at the same times each day, and avoid anything longer than a 10-minute nap during the day.
2. **Do not use your bed in the daytime** for things like watching TV, talking on the phone, or reading.
3. **Avoid** caffeine, nicotine, alcohol, heavy meals, and exercise late in the day before going to sleep.
4. **When prepared to sleep, turn off the light, and keep the room quiet and the temperature comfortable and relatively cool.** Try an electric blanket if you are cold; putting your feet outside of the blanket or turning on a fan directed toward your bed if you are hot; or wearing a sleeping mask, using earplugs, or turning on a "white noise" machine if needed.
5. **Give yourself half an hour to at most an hour to fall asleep.** If it doesn't work, evaluate whether you are calm, or anxious (even if only "background anxiety"), or ruminating.
6. **DO NOT CATASTROPHIZE.** Remind yourself that you need rest, and aim for reverie (i.e., dreaminess) and resting your brain. Sell yourself on the idea that staying awake is not a catastrophe. Do not decide to give up on sleeping for the night and get up for the "day."

IF YOU ARE CALM BUT WIDE AWAKE:

7. **Get out of bed; go to another room and read a book** or do some other activity that will not wake you up further. As you begin to get tired and/or sleepy, go back to bed.
8. **Try a light snack** (e.g., an apple).

IF YOU ARE ANXIOUS OR RUMINATING

9. **Use the cold water TIP skill. Get right back in bed and do the paced breathing TIP skill.**
    (See Distress Tolerance Handout 6: TIP Skills: Changing Your Body Chemistry.)
    Remember, if you have any medical condition, get medical approval before using cold water.
10. **Try the 9–0 meditation practice.** Breathe in deeply and breathe out slowly, saying in your mind the number 9. On the next breath out, say 8; then say 7; and so on until you breathe out saying 0. Then start over, but this time start with 8 (instead of 9) as you breathe out, followed by 7, and so on until you reach 0. Next start with 6 as you breathe out, and so on to 0. Then start with 5, then with 4, and so on until you have gone all the way down to starting with 1. (If you get lost, start over with the last number you remember.) Continue until you fall asleep.
11. **Focus on the bodily sensation** of the rumination (rumination is often escape from difficult emotional sensations).
12. **Reassure yourself** that worries in the middle of the night are just "middle-of-the-night-thinking," and that in the morning you will think and feel differently.
13. **Read an emotionally engrossing novel** for a few minutes until you feel somewhat tired. Then stop reading, close your eyes, and try to continue the novel in your head.
14. **If rumination doesn't stop,** follow these guidelines: "If it's solvable, solve it. If it is insolvable, go deep into the worry all the way to the "catastrophe"—the very worst outcome you can imagine—and then imagine coping ahead with the catastrophe.
    (See Emotion Regulation Handout 19: Build Mastery and Cope Ahead.)

If nothing else works, with eyes closed, listen to public radio (BBC, NPR, etc.) at low volume (use headphones if necessary). Public radio is a good choice for this, because there is little fluctuation in voice tone or volume.

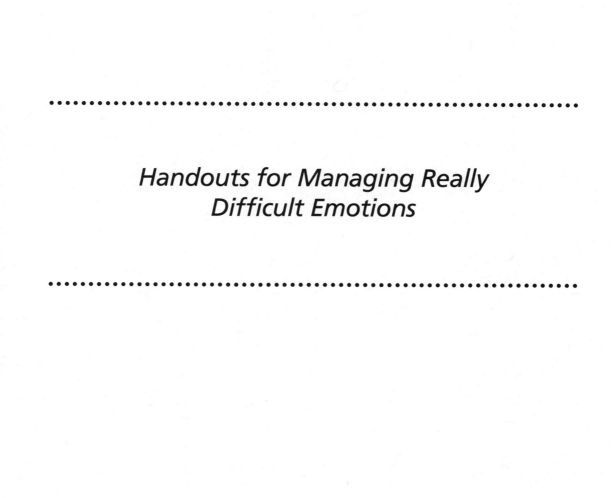

Handouts for Managing Really Difficult Emotions

Overview:
Managing Really Difficult Emotions

MINDFULNESS OF CURRENT EMOTIONS

Suppressing emotion increases suffering.

Mindfulness of current emotions is the path to emotional freedom.

MANAGING EXTREME EMOTIONS

Sometimes emotional arousal is so high that you can't use any skills, particularly if the skills are complicated or take any thought on your part.

This is a skills breakdown point.

Crisis survival skills are needed.

TROUBLESHOOTING AND REVIEW

There are many ways to change emotions.

It can be helpful to have a list of the important skills to look at when you can't remember the skills you need to regulate your emotions.

Mindfulness of Current Emotions:
Letting Go of Emotional Suffering

OBSERVE YOUR EMOTION

- Step back and just notice your emotion.
- Experience your emotion as a WAVE, coming and going.
- Now imagine surfing the emotion wave.

- Try not to BLOCK or SUPPRESS the emotion.
- Don't try to GET RID of or PUSH away the emotion.

- Don't try to KEEP the emotion around.
- Don't HOLD ON to it.
- Don't AMPLIFY it.

PRACTICE MINDFULNESS OF BODY SENSATIONS

- Notice WHERE in your body you are feeling emotional sensations.
- Experience the SENSATIONS as fully as you can.
- Observe how LONG it takes before the emotion goes down.

REMEMBER: YOU ARE NOT YOUR EMOTION

- Do not necessarily ACT on your emotion.
- Remember times when you have felt DIFFERENT.

PRACTICE LOVING YOUR EMOTION

- RESPECT your emotion.
- Do not JUDGE your emotion.
- Practice WILLINGNESS.
- Radically ACCEPT your emotion.

Managing Extreme Emotions

Follow these suggestions when emotional arousal is very **HIGH**—so extreme that your ability to use your skills breaks down.

First, observe and describe that you are at your **SKILLS BREAKDOWN POINT:**
- ❑ Your distress is extreme.
- ❑ You are overwhelmed.
- ❑ You cannot focus your mind on anything but the emotion itself.
- ❑ Your mind shuts down; your brain stops processing information.
- ❑ You cannot solve problems or use complicated skills.

Now check the facts. Are you really "falling apart" at this level of distress?

If no, **USE YOUR SKILLS.**

If yes, go to Step 1: You are at your **SKILLS BREAKDOWN POINT.**

Step 1. Use crisis survival skills to bring down your arousal:
(See Distress Tolerance Handouts 6–9a.)

- • TIP your body chemistry.
- • DISTRACT yourself from the emotional events.
- • SELF-SOOTHE through the five senses.
- • IMPROVE the moment you are in.

Step 2. Return to mindfulness of current emotions.
(See Emotion Regulation Handout 22.)

Step 3. Try other emotion regulation skills (if needed).

Troubleshooting Emotion Regulation Skills: When What You Are Doing Isn't Working

1

CHECK YOUR BIOLOGICAL SENSITIVITY

- ASK: Am I biologically more vulnerable?
  Do I have untreated physical illness or distress?
  Am I out of balance on eating, use of drugs, sleep, exercise?
  Have I taken medications as prescribed?

- WORK on your PLEASE skills.
  1. Take care of physical illness and distress.
  2. Take medications as prescribed. Check if others are needed.
  3. Try again.

2

CHECK YOUR SKILLS

- REVIEW what you have tried.
  Did you try a skill likely to be effective?
  Did you follow the skill instructions to the letter?

- WORK on your skills.
  1. Review and try other skills.
  2. Get coaching if you need it.
  3. Try again.

3

CHECK FOR REINFORCERS

- ASK: Do my emotions . . .
  COMMUNICATE an important message or influence people to do things?
  MOTIVATE me to do things I think are important?
  VALIDATE my beliefs or my identity?
  FEEL GOOD?

- IF YES:
  1. Practice interpersonal effectiveness skills to communicate.
  2. Work to find new reinforcers to motivate yourself.
  3. Practice self-validation.
  4. Do PROS AND CONS for changing emotions.
     (See Emotion Regulation Worksheet 1.)

(***continued on next page***)

4

CHECK YOUR MOOD

- ASK: Am I putting in the time and effort that solving my problem will take?

- IF NO:
    1. Do PROS AND CONS for working hard on skills.
    2. Practice RADICAL ACCEPTANCE and WILLINGNESS skills.
    3. Practice the mindfulness skills of PARTICIPATING and EFFECTIVENESS
       (See Mindfulness Handouts 4 and 5.)

5

CHECK FOR EMOTIONAL OVERLOAD

- ASK: Am I too upset to use complicated skills?

- IF YES, ask: Can the problems I am worrying about be easily solved now?
    - IF YES, do PROBLEM SOLVING.
      (See Emotion Regulation Handouts 9, 12.)
    - IF NO, practice mindfulness of CURRENT EMOTIONS.
      (See Emotion Regulation Handout 22.)

- IF your emotions are too high for you to think straight:
    - Go to TIP skills.
      (See Distress Tolerance Handout 5.)

6

CHECK FOR EMOTION MYTHS GETTING IN THE WAY

- CHECK FOR:
    Judgmental myths about emotions (e.g., "Some emotions are stupid," "There is a right way to feel in every situation")?
    Beliefs that emotions and identity are the same (e.g., "My emotions are who I am")?

- IF YES:
    1. Check the facts.
    2. Challenge myths.
    3. Practice thinking nonjudgmentally.

Review of Skills for Emotion Regulation

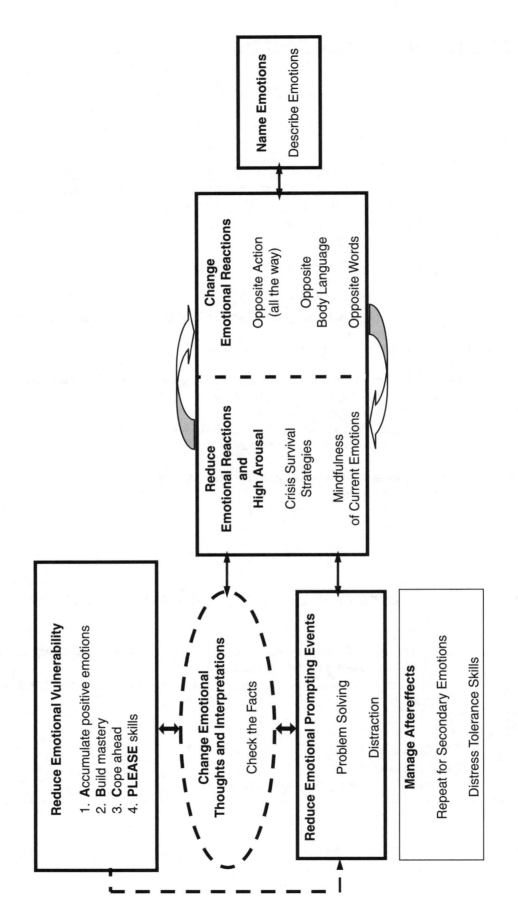

Emotion Regulation
Worksheets

(Emotion Regulation Handout 1)

Pros and Cons of Changing Emotions

Due Date: _____   Name: _____ Week Starting: _____

EMOTION NAME: _____ **INTENSITY (0–100) Before:** _____ **After:** _____

Fill this worksheet out when you are experiencing difficulties with:

- Trying to decide whether to work on changing ineffective emotions.
- Feeling willful/saying no to letting go of emotion mind.
- Deciding whether to work on reducing your emotional reactions to specific events.
- Feeling threatened whenever you think of letting go of emotions.
- Not in the mood for being effective.

When filling out this worksheet, think about these questions:

- Is living in emotion mind in your best interest (i.e., effective) or not in your best interest (i.e., ineffective)?
- Will refusing to regulate your own emotions create a new problem for you?
- Is reducing immediate high emotions likely to increase your freedom or decrease it?
- Is being attached to your emotions about a situation useful or not?
- Is working to reduce your emotion really too much work?

Make a list of the pros and cons of changing the emotion you are having difficulty with.

Make another list of the pros and cons of *not changing* your emotion.

	Stay in emotion mind, acting emotionally	Regulate emotions and emotion actions
Pros	_____ _____ _____	_____ _____ _____
Cons	Stay in emotion mind, acting emotionally _____ _____ _____	Regulate emotions and emotion actions _____ _____ _____

What did you decide to do about your emotion? _____

Is this the best decision (in Wise Mind)? _____

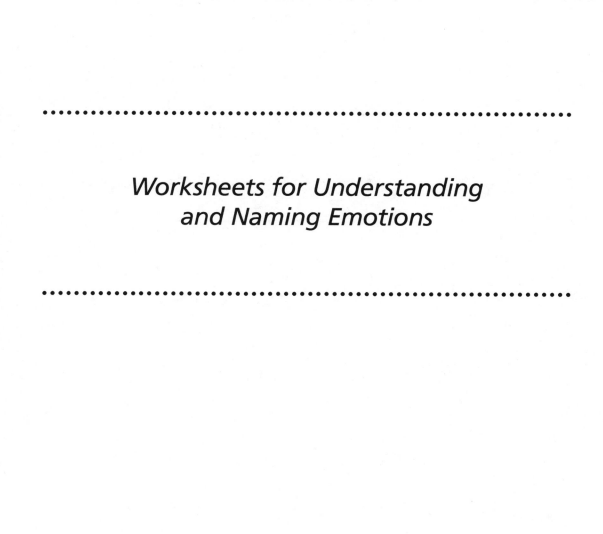

*Worksheets for Understanding
and Naming Emotions*

Figuring Out What My Emotions Are Doing for Me

Due Date: _____ Name: _____ Week Starting: _____

Select a current or recent emotional reaction and fill out as much of this sheet as you can. If the prompting event for the emotion you are working on is another emotion that occurred first (for example, feeling afraid prompted getting angry at yourself), then fill out a second worksheet for that first emotion. Write on the back of the sheet if you need more room. Remember to use your describe skills for each question.

EMOTION NAME: _____ **INTENSITY (0–100):** _____

Describe Prompting Event

What happened to prompt this emotion?

Describe Motivation to Action

What action was my emotion motivating and preparing me to do? (Was there a problem my emotion was getting me to solve, overcome, or avoid?) What function or goal did my emotion serve?

Describe Communication to Others

What was my facial expression? Posture? Gestures? Words? Actions?

What message did my emotion send to others (even if I didn't intend to send the message)?

How did my emotion influence others (even if I didn't intend to influence them)? What did others do or say as a result of my emotional expression or actions?

Describe Communication to Myself

What did my emotion say to me?

What facts could I check out to be sure the message my emotions were sending to me was correct?

What facts did I check out?

Example: Figuring Out What My Emotions Are Doing for Me

Due Date: _____ Name: _____ Week Starting: _____

Select a current or recent emotional reaction and fill out as much of this sheet as you can. If the prompting event for the emotion you are working on is another emotion that occurred first (for example, feeling afraid prompted getting angry at yourself), then fill out a second worksheet for that first emotion. Use the back of the sheet if necessary. Use describe skills for each question.

EMOTION NAME: _____*Shame and Guilt*_____**INTENSITY (0–100):** __80__

Prompting Event
What happened to prompt this emotion?
> *I left my roommate's pot on the burner and forgot about it. I destroyed it. I then threw the pot away without telling my roommate.*

Motivation to Action
What action was my emotion motivating and preparing me to do? (Was there a problem my emotion was getting me to solve, overcome, or avoid?) What function or goal did my emotion serve?
> *My emotion was motivating me to shrink away from my friend, to hide myself. It's possible that the function was to get me to change that behavior. The emotion was also functioning to get me to try to hide that I destroyed the pot.*
>
> *To influence my friend to stop being mad at me.*

Communication to Others
What was my facial expression? Posture? Gestures? Words? Actions?
> *My eyes were looking down. My lips were turned down. I was slouched slightly and turned slightly away from my friend. I did not say anything. I put my hands on my forehead.*

What message did my emotion send to others (even if I didn't intend to send the message)?
> *I think my friend realized that I felt bad.*

How did my emotion influence others (even if I didn't intend to influence them)? What did others do or say as a result of my emotional expression or actions?
> *My friend tried to get me to talk. I think it influenced her to stop yelling at me and be more kind.*

Communication to Myself
What did my emotion say to me?
> *It was wrong to do what I did. I feel badly about it because I disappointed my friend. I have really messed this up and now she will never trust or like me.*

What facts could I check out to be sure the message my emotions were sending to me was correct?
> *I could ask myself if what I did would get me kicked out of my house/friendship. I could try to figure out if what I did crossed my own wise/clear mind, moral code, values. I could ask her: Have I destroyed the relationship? Is she going to kick me out? Stop spending time with me? I could also ask what I can do that would help her to trust me again.*

What facts did I check out?
> *I felt bad about burning the pot—but it wasn't a moral code or values issue yet until I tried to hide that I had done it. That behavior did go against my Wise Mind. I asked my roommate if she hated me now and she said no. I asked if there was anything I could do to fix the situation, and she asked me to buy a new pot, and I did.*

Emotion Diary

Name: _____   Week Starting: _____

Record an emotion (either the strongest emotion of the day, the longest-lasting one, or the one that was the most painful or gave you the most trouble). Analyze that emotion. Fill out an Observing and Describing Emotions worksheet (Emotion Regulation Worksheet 4 or 4a) if necessary, plus this diary sheet.

Emotions	Motivate		Communicate to others		Communicate to me	
Emotion name	What did my emotion motivate me to do (i.e., what goal did my emotion serve)?	How was my emotion expressed to others (my nonverbal appearance, my words, my actions)?	What message did my emotion express to others?	What was the effect of my emotion on others?	What was my emotion saying to me?	How did I check the facts?

Example: Emotion Diary

Due Date: _____ Name: _____ Week Starting: _____

Record an emotion (either the strongest emotion of the day, the longest-lasting one, or the one that was the most painful or gave you the most trouble). Analyze that emotion. Fill out an Observing and Describing Emotions worksheet (Emotion Regulation Worksheet 4 or 4a) if necessary, plus this diary sheet.

Emotions	Motivate	Communicate to others			Communicate to me	
Emotion name	What did my emotion motivate me to do (i.e., what goal did my emotion serve)?	How was my emotion expressed to others (my nonverbal appearance, my words, my actions)?	What message did my emotion express to others?	What was the effect of my emotion on others?	What was my emotion saying to me?	How did I check the facts?
Fear/ anxiety	Not to go to skills training group.	I did not go to group.	That group was not important to me.	(1) They called to encourage me to come. (2) They wonder if I am committed. (3) They might be concerned.	That group is unsafe.	I didn't. I could have evaluated if my life, health, or well-being was in danger. I could have done pros and cons of going to group.
Shame	To keep to myself, to not draw attention to myself. I wanted to go home from the office party at work.	I didn't make much eye contact, I didn't say much or initiate conversation, or do anything to attract attention.	There are several possibilities: (1) I want to be left alone. (2) I am feeling bad.	Most everyone at work left me alone. One person tried to talk to me but gave up.	That I was uninteresting, a failure with nothing to contribute.	I tried to recall times when people have listened to me. I tried to talk to others and notice if they seemed interested.
Sadness	Withdraw. Isolate. Cry.	My expression was downcast. My mouth turned down. I was tearful. I told someone I was sad.	That I was sad.	(1) My boyfriend approached me, soothed me, and invited me to sit with him. (2) Some people avoided me.	I am so sad. I am alone. No one cares.	I reached out and noticed if someone responded. I thought about a time when I did not feel sad.

Myths about Emotions

Due Date: _____   Name: _____ Week Starting: _____

For each myth, write down a challenge that makes sense to you. Although the one already written may make a lot of sense, try to come up with another one or rewrite the one there in your own words.

1. There is a right way to feel in every situation.
   Challenge: Every person responds differently to a situation. There is no correct or right way.
   My challenge: _____

2. Letting others know that I am feeling bad is a weakness.
   Challenge: Letting others know that I am feeling bad is a healthy form of communication.
   My challenge: _____

3. Negative feelings are bad and destructive.
   Challenge: Negative feelings are natural responses. They help me to create a better understanding of the situation.
   My challenge: _____

4. Being emotional means being out of control.
   Challenge: Being emotional means being a normal human being.
   My challenge: _____

5. Some emotions are stupid.
   Challenge: Every emotion indicates how I am feeling in a certain situation. All emotions are useful to help me understand what I am experiencing.
   My challenge: _____

6. All painful emotions are a result of a bad attitude.
   Challenge: All painful emotions are natural responses to something.
   My challenge: _____

7. If others don't approve of my feelings, I obviously shouldn't feel the way I do.
   Challenge: I have every right to feel the way I do, regardless of what other people think.
   My challenge: _____

8. Other people are the best judges of how I am feeling.
   Challenge: I am the best judge of how I feel. Other people can only guess how I feel.
   My challenge: _____

9. Painful emotions are not important and should be ignored.
   Challenge: Painful emotions can be warning signs telling me that a situation I am in is not good.
   My challenge: _____

10. Extreme emotions get you a lot further than trying to regulate your emotions.
    Challenge: Extreme emotions can often cause trouble for me and for other people. If an emotion is not effective, emotion regulation is a good idea.
    My challenge: _____

(*continued on next page*)

11. Creativity requires intense, often out-of-control emotions.
Challenge: I can be in control of my emotions and be creative.

My challenge: _____

12. Drama is cool.
Challenge: I can be dramatic and regulate my emotions.

My challenge: _____

13. It is inauthentic to try to change my emotions.
Challenge: Change is itself authentic; it is part of life.

My challenge: _____

14. Emotional truth is what counts, not factual truth.
Challenge: Both emotional feeling and facts matter.

My challenge: _____

15. People should do whatever they feel like doing.
Challenge: Doing what I feel like doing can be ineffective.

My challenge: _____

16. Acting on your emotions is the mark of a truly free individual.
Challenge: The truly free person can regulate emotions.

My challenge: _____

17. My emotions are who I am.
Challenge: Emotions are partly but not completely who I am.

My challenge: _____

18. My emotions are why people love me.
Challenge: People will still love me if I regulate my emotions.

My challenge: _____

19. Emotions can just happen for no reason.
Challenge: All things in the universe are caused.

My challenge: _____

20. Emotions should always be trusted.
Challenge: Emotions should sometimes be trusted.

My challenge: _____

21. Other myth: _____
Challenge:

My challenge: _____

Observing and Describing Emotions

Due Date: _____ Name: _____

Week Starting: _____

Select a current or recent emotional reaction, and fill out as much of this sheet as you can. If the prompting event for the emotion you are working on is another emotion that occurred first (e.g., fear prompted anger at yourself), then fill out a second worksheet for the first emotion. Use Emotion Regulation Handout 6 for ideas. Write on the back of this sheet if you need more room.

Vulnerability Factors: What happened before to make me vulnerable to the prompting event? Tell the story up to the event.

_____
_____

Emotion Name: _____

Intensity (0–100) _____

Expressions

Face and Body Language: What is or was my facial expression? Posture? Gestures?

_____

Expression with Words: What I SAID

_____

Actions: What I DID

_____

Biological Changes

Face and Body Changes and Experiences: What am I or was I feeling in my face and body?

_____

Action Urges

What do I or did I feel like doing? What do I or did I want to say?

_____

Interpretation of Event: Thoughts, beliefs, assumptions, appraisals?

_____

Prompting Event: What set off the emotion? What happened in the few minutes right before the emotion started? Just the facts!

_____

Aftereffects: Emotions, behavior, thoughts, etc.?

_____

Observing and Describing Emotions

Due Date: _____ Name: _____ Week Starting: _____

Select a current or recent emotional reaction, and fill out as much of this sheet as you can. If the prompting event for the emotion you are working on is another emotion that occurred first (e.g., fear prompted anger at yourself), then fill out a second worksheet for the first emotion. Use Emotion Regulation Handout 6 for ideas. Write on the back of this sheet if you need more room.

EMOTION NAME: _____ **INTENSITY (0–100):** _____

PROMPTING EVENT for my emotion (who, what, when, where): What set off the emotion?

_____

_____

VULNERABILITY FACTORS: What happened before that made me vulnerable to the prompting event?

_____

_____

INTERPRETATIONS (beliefs, assumptions, appraisals) of the situation:

_____

_____

FACE and BODY CHANGES and EXPERIENCES: What was I feeling in my face and body?

_____

_____

ACTION URGES: What did I feel like doing? What did I want to say?

_____

_____

FACE and BODY LANGUAGE: What was my facial expression? Posture? Gestures?

_____

_____

What I SAID in the situation (be specific):

_____

_____

What I DID in the situation (be specific):

_____

_____

What AFTEREFFECTS did the emotion have on me (my state of mind, other emotions, behavior, thoughts, memory, body, etc.)?

_____

_____

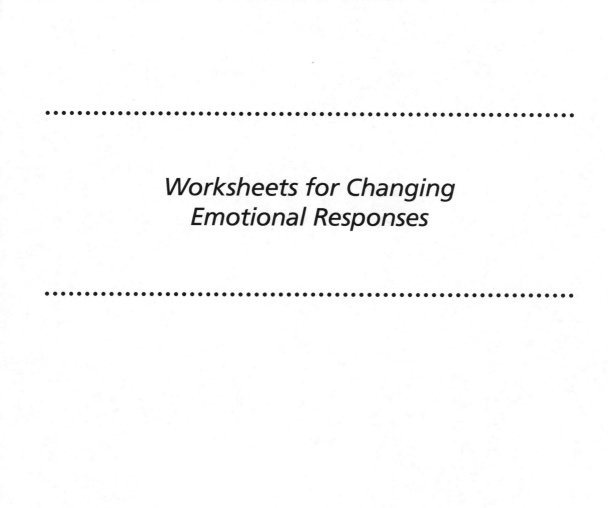

Worksheets for Changing Emotional Responses

Check the Facts

Due Date: _____   Name: _____ Week Starting: _____

It is hard to problem-solve an emotional situation if you don't have your facts straight. You must know what the problem is before you can solve it. This worksheet helps you figure out whether it is the event that is causing your emotion, your interpretation of the event, or both. Use your mindfulness skills of observing and describing. Observe the facts, and then describe the facts you have observed.

Step 1

Ask: **What emotion do I want to change?**

EMOTION NAME: _____ INTENSITY (0–100) Before: _____ After: _____

Step 2

Ask: **What is the PROMPTING EVENT for my emotional reaction?**

DESCRIBE THE PROMPTING EVENT: What happened that led you to have this emotion? Who did what to whom? What led up to what? What is it about this event that is a problem for you? Be very specific in your answers.

_____

_____

CHECK THE FACTS!

Look for extremes and judgments in the way you are describing the prompting event.

REWRITE the facts, if necessary, to be more accurate.

Facts →

_____

_____

Step 3

Ask: **What are my INTERPRETATIONS (thoughts, beliefs, etc.) about the facts?** What am I assuming? Am I adding my own interpretations to the description of the prompting event?

_____

_____

CHECK THE FACTS!

List as many *other* possible interpretations of the facts as you can.

_____

_____

REWRITE the facts, if necessary. Try to check the accuracy of your interpretations. If you can't check the facts, write out a likely or a useful (i.e., effective) interpretation.

Facts →

_____

_____

*(**continued on next page**)*

Step 4

Ask: **Am I assuming a THREAT?** What is the THREAT? What about this event or situation is threatening to me? What worrisome consequences or outcomes am I expecting?

_____

_____

_____

CHECK THE FACTS!

List as many _other_ possible outcomes as you can, given the facts.

_____

_____

REWRITE the facts if needed. Try to check the accuracy of your expectations. If you can't check out probable outcomes, write out a likely noncatastrophic outcome to expect.

_____

Facts →

_____

_____

Step 5

Ask: **What's the CATASTROPHE, even if the outcome I am worrying about does occur?** Describe in detail the worst outcome I can reasonably expect.

_____

_____

DESCRIBE WAYS TO COPE if the worst does happen.

_____

_____

_____

Step 6

ASK: **Does my emotion (or its intensity or duration) FIT THE FACTS?**
(0 = not at all to 5 = I am certain): _____

If you are unsure whether your emotion or your emotional intensity fits the facts (for example, you give a score of 2, 3, or 4), keep checking the facts. Be as creative as you can be; ask others for their opinions; or do an experiment to see if your predictions or interpretations are correct.

Describe what you did to check the facts:

_____

_____

_____

Figuring Out How to Change Unwanted Emotions

Due Date: _____ Name: _____ Week Starting: _____

Once you have checked the facts, use this worksheet to help you figure out what to do next. Before you can figure out what to change, you have to decide whether acting on your emotion is effective in the situation you are in (and whether the emotion is one you actually want to change). (If you are not sure whether you want to change it or not, go back to Emotion Regulation Worksheet 1 and do pros and cons.) In the flow chart below, circle Yes or No at each level, and then select the skill that fits your situation best.

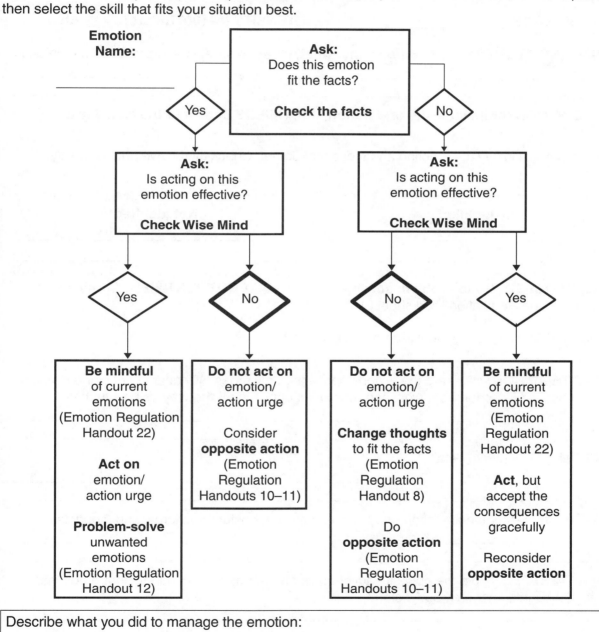

Emotion Name:

_____

Ask: Does this emotion fit the facts?

Check the facts

Yes → **Ask:** Is acting on this emotion effective? **Check Wise Mind**

No → **Ask:** Is acting on this emotion effective? **Check Wise Mind**

Yes → **Be mindful** of current emotions (Emotion Regulation Handout 22)

Act on emotion/ action urge

Problem-solve unwanted emotions (Emotion Regulation Handout 12)

No → **Do not act on** emotion/ action urge

Consider **opposite action** (Emotion Regulation Handouts 10–11)

No → **Do not act on** emotion/ action urge

Change thoughts to fit the facts (Emotion Regulation Handout 8)

Do **opposite action** (Emotion Regulation Handouts 10–11)

Yes → **Be mindful** of current emotions (Emotion Regulation Handout 22)

Act, but accept the consequences gracefully

Reconsider **opposite action**

Describe what you did to manage the emotion:

Opposite Action to Change Emotions

Due Date: _____ Name: _____ Week Starting: _____

Select a current or recent emotional reaction that you find painful or want to change. Figure out if the emotion fits the facts. If it does not, then notice your action urges; figure out what would be opposite actions; and then do the opposite actions. Remember to practice opposite action *all the way*. Describe what happened.

EMOTION NAME: _____ **INTENSITY (0–100) Before:** _____ **After:** _____

PROMPTING EVENT for my emotion (who, what, when, where): What prompted the emotion.

_____

_____

IS MY EMOTION (or its intensity or duration) JUSTIFIED? Does it fit the facts? Is it effective?

List the facts that justify the emotion and those that do not. Check the answer that is mostly correct.

Justified	Not justified
_____	_____
_____	_____

❑ **JUSTIFIED: Go to problem solving** (Emotion Regulation Worksheet 8) ❑ **NOT JUSTIFIED: Continue**

ACTION URGES: What do I feel like doing or saying?

_____

OPPOSITE ACTION: What are the actions opposite to my urges? What am I not doing because of my emotions? Describe both *what* and *how* to act opposite **all the way** in the situation.

_____

_____

WHAT I did: Describe in detail.

_____

_____

HOW I did it: Describe body language, facial expression, posture, gestures, and thoughts.

_____

_____

What **AFTEREFFECT** did the opposite action have on me (my state of mind, other emotions, behavior, thoughts, memory, body, etc.)?

_____

_____

Problem Solving to Change Emotions

Due Date: _____ Name: _____ Week Starting: _____

Select a prompting event that triggers a painful emotion. Select an event that can be changed. Turn the event into a problem to be solved. Follow the steps below and describe what happened.

EMOTION NAME: _____ **INTENSITY (0–100) Before:** _____ **After:** _____

1. **WHAT IS THE PROBLEM?** Describe the problem prompting your emotions. What makes the situation a problem?

   _____

   _____

   _____

2. **CHECK THE FACTS TO MAKE SURE YOU HAVE THE RIGHT PROBLEM.** Describe what you did to be sure of your facts.
   (See Emotion Regulation Worksheet 6 if you need help.)

   _____

   _____

   REWRITE the problem if needed to stick with the facts.

   _____

   _____

3. **WHAT IS A REALISTIC SHORT-TERM GOAL OF YOUR PROBLEM SOLVING**? What has to happen for you to think you have made progress?

   _____

   _____

   _____

4. **BRAINSTORM SOLUTIONS:** List as many solutions and coping strategies as you can think of. DON'T EVALUATE!

   _____

   _____

   _____

   _____

   _____

*(**continued on next page**)*

5. WHICH TWO IDEAS LOOK BEST (are most likely to meet your goal, are possible to do)?

1. _____ 2. _____

	Solution 1	Solution 2
PROS	_____ _____ _____ _____	_____ _____ _____ _____
	Solution 1	**Solution 2**
CONS	_____ _____ _____ _____	_____ _____ _____ _____

6. CHOOSE the solution to try; list the steps needed; check the steps you do and how well they work.

Step	Describe	✓ Done	What happened?
1.	_____	_____	_____
2.	_____	_____	_____
3.	_____	_____	_____
4.	_____	_____	_____
5.	_____	_____	_____
6.	_____	_____	_____
7.	_____	_____	_____

7. DID YOU REACH YOUR GOAL? If so, describe. If not, what can you do next?

_____

_____

IS THERE NOW A NEW PROBLEM TO BE SOLVED? If yes, describe, and problem-solve again.

_____

_____

_____

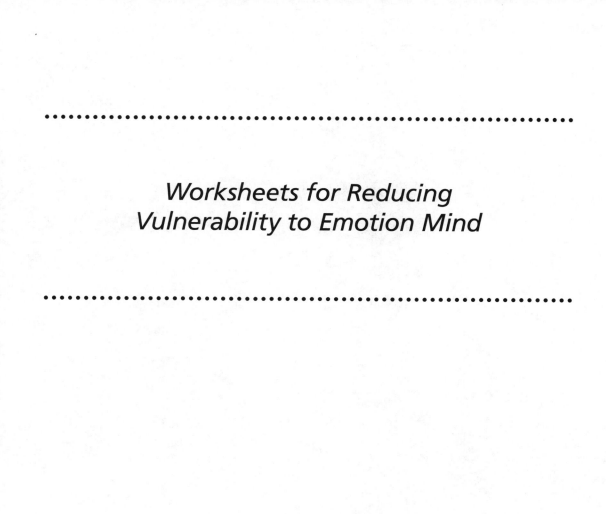

*Worksheets for Reducing
Vulnerability to Emotion Mind*

Steps for Reducing Vulnerability to Emotion Mind

Due Date: _____ Name: _____ Week Starting: _____

For each emotion regulation skill, note whether you used it during the week, and describe what you did. Write on the back of this sheet if you need more room.

A

ACCUMULATE POSITIVE EMOTIONS: SHORT TERM
INCREASED daily pleasant activities (circle):   M   T   W   Th   F   S   Sun

Describe: _____

_____

_____

ACCUMULATE POSITIVE EMOTIONS: LONG TERM; BUILDING A LIFE WORTH LIVING

VALUES considered in deciding what goals to work on (see Emotion Regulation Handout 18):

_____

_____

LONG-TERM GOALS worked on (describe): _____

_____

_____

AVOIDED AVOIDING (describe): _____

_____

_____

MINDFULNESS OF POSITIVE EXPERIENCES WHEN THEY OCCURRED
Focused (and refocused) attention on positive experiences: _____

Distracted from worries if they showed up: _____

B

BUILD MASTERY
Scheduled activities to build a sense of accomplishment (circle):   M   T   W   Th   F   S   Sun

Describe: _____

_____

Actually did something difficult, **BUT** possible (circle):   M   T   W   Th   F   S   Sun

Describe: _____

_____

C

COPE AHEAD
Describe a situation that prompts unwanted emotions (fill out Steps 1 and 2 of checking the facts on Emotion Regulation Worksheet 5 if necessary):

_____

_____

Way that I imagined coping effectively (describe): _____

_____

_____

Way that I imagined coping with new problems that might arise (describe): _____

_____

_____

(***continued on next page***)

PLEASE Skills

Have I . . .

Treated PhysicaL illness? _____

_____

Balanced Eating? _____

_____

Avoided mood-Altering substances? _____

_____

Balanced Sleep? _____

_____

Exercised? _____

_____

Pleasant Events Diary

Due Date: _____ Name: _____ Week Starting: _____

Accumulating pleasant events can take planning. For each day of the week, write down at least one pleasant activity or event that is possible for you. In the next column, write down for each day the pleasant event or activity that you actually engaged in. Fill out an Observing and Describing Emotions worksheet (Emotion Regulation Worksheet 4 or 4a) if necessary, plus this diary sheet.

Day of week	Pleasant event(s) planned	Pleasant event(s) I actually did	Mindfulness of pleasant event (0–5)	Letting go of worries (0–5)	Pleasant experience (0–100)	Comments

Getting from Values to Specific Action Steps

Due Date: _____ Name: _____ Week Starting: _____

STEP 1. AVOID AVOIDING. Rate degree you have avoided working on building a life worth living:

In the past (____) Now (____) (0 = no avoidance, 100 = avoided completely even thinking about it)

Check reasons for avoiding: ❑ Hopelessness ❑ Willfulness ❑ Too hard ❑ Other: _____

> Use your cope-ahead skills, and write out a plan for getting yourself to avoid avoiding.

STEP 2. IDENTIFY VALUES THAT ARE IMPORTANT TO YOU. What is most important to you? Review Emotion Regulation Handout 18 for ideas. Make a list of several of your most important values.

MY IMPORTANT VALUES: _____

_____

STEP 3. IDENTIFY ONE IMPORTANT LIFE VALUE OR PRIORITY TO WORK ON NOW.

Long-term goals depend on Wise Mind values and priorities. What values in your life need more work now?

Make a list of two of the **most important** values in your life that are important things for you to work on right now.

	Importance	Priority
VALUE: _____	( )	( )
VALUE: _____	( )	( )

Rate the importance of each value for a "life worth living" to you (1 = a little important, 5 = extremely important). Then rate how important it is to work on this value NOW (1 = low priority, 5 = very high priority).

REFINE YOUR CHOICES. Review your list and ratings above and the value you have chosen to work on now. **CHECK THE FACTS.** Make sure that what you think are values and priorities are in fact YOUR values and priorities—not the values others have, the values others think you should have, or old internal "tapes" of values you learned but no longer really believe in. Rewrite your list if you need to.

CHOOSE A VALUE TO WORK ON NOW. Pick the value that is either the most important to you or is your highest priority to work on right now. (If you have more than one value that is a high priority to work on right now, fill out another worksheet for that value.)

VALUE TO WORK ON NOW: _____

(*continued on next page*)

STEP 4. IDENTIFY A FEW GOALS RELATED TO THIS VALUE.

List two or three **different goals** related to this value. Be specific. What can you do to make this value a part of your life? (If you have trouble thinking of goals, brainstorm as many goals as you can think of that might be related, and then choose those most related to your values.)

GOAL: _____

GOAL: _____

GOAL: _____

STEP 5. CHOOSE ONE GOAL TO WORK ON NOW.

Select one goal that is reasonable to work on *now.* If one goal has to be accomplished before other goals can be worked on, choose that one as your working-on goal. Be specific. If you want to work on more than one goal at a time, fill out two worksheets.

Goal to work on: _____

STEP 6. IDENTIFY SMALL ACTION STEPS TOWARD YOUR GOAL.

Break down the goal into lots of small steps that you can do. Each small step is a subgoal on the way to your overall goal. List action steps that will get you closer to your goal. If you can't think of any steps, try brainstorming ideas. Write down whatever comes to your mind.

If you start to feel *overwhelmed* because a step looks too big, erase it and break it down into smaller steps you think you can actually do. Rewrite your list if you need to so that the steps you think you can do are included. Put in the order that you think you should do them. If you start to feel *overwhelmed* because there are too many steps, stop writing new steps and focus on just one step.

Action Step 1: _____

Action Step 2: _____

Action Step 3: _____

Action Step 4: _____

STEP 7. TAKE ONE ACTION STEP NOW. Describe what you did: _____

_____

_____

Describe what happened next: _____

_____

_____

(*continued on next page*)

REMEMBER: ATTEND TO RELATIONSHIPS

Attending to relationships (Group A on Emotion Regulation Handout 18) and being part of a group (Group B) are important to just about everyone. If you did not choose a value from one of these groups, review them to see if one of these first 10 values is an important one for you to work on. If you choose one, write it down and then, after working on it, fill out the rest of the worksheet.

Describe the relationship or relationship problem you want to work on: _____

_____

_____

What goal can you work on now? _____

_____

What small action steps will help you reach your goal?

Action Step 1: _____

Action Step 2: _____

Action Step 3: _____

Action Step 4: _____

TAKE ONE ACTION STEP NOW. Describe what you did: _____

_____

Describe what happened next: _____

_____

Getting from Values to Specific Action Steps

Due Date: _____ Name: _____ Week Starting: _____

Once you have figured out your values, the next step is to decide on specific things you can do or achieve (goals) that will make your life more in line with your values. Once you have goals, you can figure out what action steps are necessary to achieve the goal.

> **Example:** **VALUE:** Be part of a group.
>
> Possible **GOALS:**
> - Reconnect with old friends.
> - Get a more social job.
> - Join a club.
>
> Pick one **GOAL** to work on right now.
> - Join a club.
>
> Figure out a few **ACTION STEPS** that will move me toward my goal.
> - Look for clubs on craigslist.
> - Go to the bookstore by my house and ask about book groups.
> - Join an interactive online game or chat room.

1. Pick one of your **VALUES:**

_____

2. Identify three **GOALS:**

_____

_____

_____

3. Circle one **GOAL** to work on right now.

4. Identify **ACTION STEPS** you can take right now to move closer to this **GOAL.**

_____

_____

5. Take one **ACTION STEP** now. Describe what you did:

_____

_____

Describe what happened next: _____

_____

Diary of Daily Actions on Values and Priorities

Due Date: _____ Name: _____ Week Starting: _____

This diary is for tracking your progress in reaching your goals and living according to your own values. You can either fill out one page for each value or goal you are working on, or you can fill it out every day no matter what goal you are working on that day. Remember to be very specific. Check Emotion Regulation Worksheet 11 or 11a for your list of important values and goals.

Day	Value What value am I working on?	Goal What is my goal related to this value?	Value and Priority Actions Today What action did I do today to achieve this goal? (Be specific.)	Next Step What will my next action be to achieve this goal? (Be specific.)

Build Mastery and Cope Ahead

Due Date: _____ Name: _____ Week Starting: _____

In the far left column, put down the days of the week. Then write plans for practicing mastery in the first column under "Build Mastery." At the end of the day, write in the second column what you actually did to increase your sense of mastery. Under "Cope Ahead," describe a problem situation in the first column, and then describe in the second column how you imagined coping skillfully. Also, check whether it helped.

Build Mastery		
Day	Activities planned for building mastery	Activities I actually did for building mastery

Cope Ahead	
Future problem situation	How I imagined coping effectively (describe)
1.	Helpful? ☐ YES ☐ NO
2.	Helpful? ☐ YES ☐ NO

Putting ABC Skills Together Day by Day

Due Date: _____   Name: _____   Week Starting: _____

This worksheet is for tracking your planned ABC tasks throughout each day. At night or first thing in the morning, write down what you plan to do that day; as you go or at the end of the day, write down what you actually did. Over time, you will find that you can do more and more of what you plan, and as you do that you will find your vulnerability to negative emotions going down.

Rate your negative mood or emotions at start of day (0–100): _____   And negative mood or emotions at end of day (0–100): _____

Daytime Hours	PLANNED ACTIVITIES			WHAT I ACTUALLY DID		
	<u>A</u>ccumulate Positive Emotions	Action to <u>B</u>uild Mastery	<u>C</u>ope-Ahead Task	<u>A</u>ccumulate Positive Emotions	Action to <u>B</u>uild Mastery	<u>C</u>ope-Ahead Task
Before 8 A.M.						
8 A.M. to 12 noon						
12 noon to 4 P.M.						
4 P.M. to 8 P.M.						
After 8 P.M.						
Total Number of Activities						

Practicing PLEASE Skills

Due Date: _____ Name: _____ Week Starting: _____

In the left column, put down the days of the week. Then write down what you did to practice each of the PLEASE skills. At the bottom of each column, check whether practicing this skill was helpful during the week.

Day	Describe treating Physical illness	Describe balanced Eating efforts	List mood-Altering substances used	Hours of Sleep (time to bed; time up)	Describe Exercise (hours and/or minutes)
	Helpful? ☐ YES ☐ NO	Helpful? ☐ YES ☐ NO	Helpful? ☐ YES ☐ NO	Helpful? ☐ YES ☐ NO	Helpful? ☐ YES ☐ NO

Target Nightmare Experience Forms (Set of 3)

Due Date: _____   Name: _____ Week Starting: _____

In the space provided below, describe the distressing dream in as many details as possible. Include sensory descriptions (sights, smells, sounds, tastes, etc.). Note the feelings, images, and thoughts associated with this dream, including assumptions about yourself. Be as specific as possible. Note when the dream begins and when it ends. (Use the back of this sheet if necessary.)

In my dream, _____

_____

_____

_____

_____

_____

_____

_____

_____

_____

_____

_____

_____

_____

_____

_____

_____

_____

_____

_____

_____

(*continued on next page*)

Changed Dream Experience Form

Due Date: _____ Name: _____ Week Starting: _____

In the space provided below, describe the changed dream in as many details as possible. Include sensory descriptions (sights, smells, sounds, tastes, etc.). Please note the feelings, images, and thoughts associated with this dream, including assumptions about yourself. Be as specific as possible. Be sure the change you put in occurs *before* anything traumatic or bad happens to you or others in the nightmare. Note when the dream begins and when it ends. (Use the back of this sheet if necessary.)

In my dream, _____

_____

_____

_____

_____

_____

_____

_____

_____

_____

_____

_____

_____

_____

_____

_____

_____

_____

_____

_____

_____

_____

_____

_____

_____

_____

_____

(*continued on next page*)

Dream Rehearsal and Relaxation Record

Due Date: _____ Name: _____ Week Starting: _____

In the left column, put down the days of the week. Then write down what you did to practice dream rehearsal and relaxation during the week. In the morning write down the intensity of your nightmare. (Put a 0 if you did not have the nightmare.) Continue practicing until you do not have the nightmare again.

Day	Describe daytime visual rehearsal and relaxation	Negative emotion intensity (0–100)	Describe daytime visual rehearsal and relaxation	Negative emotion intensity (0–100)	Describe daytime visual rehearsal and relaxation	Nightmare intensity (0–100)
		Start: ___ End: ___		Start: ___ End: ___		
		Start: ___ End: ___		Start: ___ End: ___		
		Start: ___ End: ___		Start: ___ End: ___		
		Start: ___ End: ___		Start: ___ End: ___		
		Start: ___ End: ___		Start: ___ End: ___		
		Start: ___ End: ___		Start: ___ End: ___		
		Start: ___ End: ___		Start: ___ End: ___		

Sleep Hygiene Practice Sheet

Due Date: _____ Name: _____ Week Starting: _____

In the far left column, put down the days of the week. Then put times/hours in bed, and what you did in the 4 hours before bed, in the next three columns. Along with describing the strategies you used, please rate your degree of rumination before and after using skills. Write in 0 if you had no rumination. Finally, rate the overall usefulness of your strategies.

Day	Time to bed/ time up	Hours/ minutes in bed during the day	Food, drink, exercise within 4 hours of bed	Starting emotion/ rumination intensity (0–100)	Describe strategies used to get to sleep (or back to sleep)	Ending emotion/ rumination intensity (0–100)	Usefulness of strategies (0–100)
	_____ _____	Hrs: ____ Min: ____					
	_____ _____	Hrs: ____ Min: ____					
	_____ _____	Hrs: ____ Min: ____					
	_____ _____	Hrs: ____ Min: ____					
	_____ _____	Hrs: ____ Min: ____					
	_____ _____	Hrs: ____ Min: ____					
	_____ _____	Hrs: ____ Min: ____					

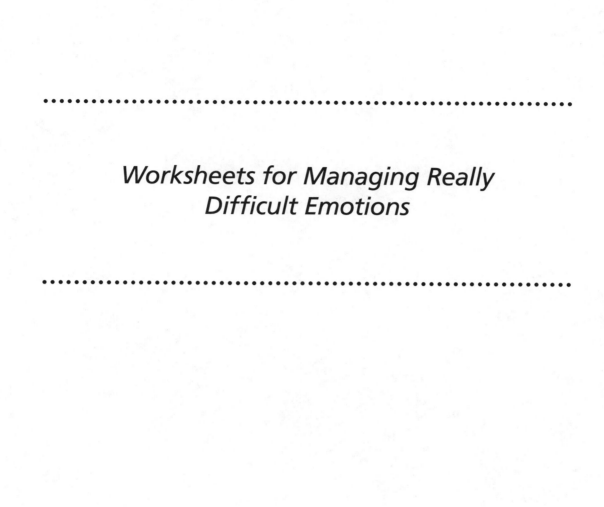

Worksheets for Managing Really Difficult Emotions

Mindfulness of Current Emotions

Due Date: _____ Name: _____ Week Starting: _____

EMOTION NAME: _____ **INTENSITY (0–100) Before:** _____ **After:** _____

Describe situation that prompts emotion. (Fill out Steps 1 and 2 on Emotion Regulation Worksheet 5, if necessary.)

When emotional intensity is extreme, go to **CRISIS SURVIVAL SKILLS first** and fill out Distress Tolerance Worksheets 2–6. With any emotion, high or low, practice radical acceptance with **MINDFULNESS OF CURRENT EMOTIONS.**

Check off any of the following that you did:

❑ Stepped back and just noticed the emotions I was experiencing.
❑ Experienced the emotion as waves, coming and going on the beach.
❑ Let go of judgments about my emotions.
❑ Noticed where in my body I was feeling the emotional sensations.

❑ Paid attention to the physical sensations of the emotions as much as I could.
❑ Observed how long it took the emotion to go away.
❑ Reminded myself that being critical of emotions does not work.
❑ Practiced willingness to have unwelcome emotions.
❑ Imagined my emotions as clouds in the sky, coming and going.
❑ Just noticed the action urge that went with my emotion.

❑ Got myself to avoid acting on my emotion.
❑ Reminded myself of times when I have felt different.
❑ Practiced radically accepting my emotion.
❑ Tried to love my emotions.

Other: _____

Comments and descriptions of experiences:

Troubleshooting Emotion Regulation Skills

Due Date: _____   Name: _____   Week Starting: _____

When you just can't get your skills to work, try doing this worksheet to see if you can figure out what is going wrong. Check off each box in order, follow the directions and keep going until you find a solution.

EMOTION NAME: _____ **INTENSITY (0–100) Before:** _____ **After:** _____

List the skill you were trying to use that did not seem to help: _____

1. **Am I biologically more vulnerable?**
   - ❑ **NO:** Go to next question.
      - ❑ **NOT SURE:** Review the PLEASE skills. *(See Emotion Regulation Handout 20.)*
      - ❑ **YES:** Work on PLEASE skills. *(See Emotion Regulation Worksheet 14.)* Consider medication.
         Did this help? ❑ *No (Go to next question)* ❑ *Yes (Fabulous)* ❑ *Didn't do it*

2. **Did I use the skill correctly? Check out the instructions.**
   - ❑ **YES:** Go to next question.
      - ❑ **NOT SURE:** Reread the instructions or get coaching. TRY AGAIN.
         Did this help? ❑ *No (Go to next question)* ❑ *Yes (Fabulous)* ❑ *Didn't do it*

3. **Are my emotions being reinforced (and maybe I don't really want to change them)?**
   - ❑ **NO:** Go to next question.
      - ❑ **NOT SURE:** Review Emotion Regulation Handout 3/Worksheets 2, 2a.
      - ❑ **YES:** Do a PROS and CONS for changing emotions. *(See Emotion Regulation Worksheet 1.)*
         Did this help? ❑ *No (Go to next question)* ❑ *Yes (Fabulous)* ❑ *Didn't do it*

4. **Am I putting in the time and effort that emotion regulation takes?**
   - ❑ **YES:** Continue practicing.
      - ❑ **NO:** Practice radical acceptance and willingness. *(See Distress Tolerance Handouts 11b and 13.)*
         Practice participating and effectiveness. *(See Mindfulness Handouts 4 and 5.)*
         Use problem solving to find the time to work on skills. *(See Emotion Regulation Worksheet 8.)*
         Did this help? ❑ *No (Go to next question)* ❑ *Yes (Fabulous)* ❑ *Didn't do it*

5. **Are my emotions too extreme right now for skills? Am I going around in so many circles that I have fallen into the emotional sea of dyscontrol?**
   - ❑ **NO:** Go to next question.
      - ❑ **YES:** If possible *now*, solve the problem. *(See Emotion Regulation Handout 12, Worksheet 9.)*
         If not possible, *attend to physical sensations. (See Emotion Regulation Handout 22.)*
         If too extreme for skills, go to TIP skills. *(See Distress Tolerance Handout 5.)*
         Did this help? ❑ *No (Go to next question)* ❑ *Yes (Fabulous)* ❑ *Didn't do it*

6. **Are myths about emotions and emotion regulation getting in my way?**
   - ❑ **NO.**
      - ❑ **YES:** Practice nonjudgmentalness. Check the facts and challenge the myths.
         Did this help? ❑ *No* ❑ *Yes (Fabulous)* ❑ *Didn't do it*

DISTRESS TOLERANCE SKILLS

Introduction to Handouts and Worksheets

Distress tolerance is the ability to tolerate and survive crises without making things worse. The ability to tolerate and accept distress is essential for two reasons. First, pain and distress are part of life; they cannot be entirely avoided or removed. The inability to accept this immutable fact increases pain and suffering. Second, distress tolerance, at least over the short run, is part of any attempt to change yourself. Otherwise, efforts to escape pain and distress will interfere with your efforts to establish desired changes. There are two main sets of handouts and worksheets for distress tolerance skills: **Crisis Survival Skills** and **Reality Acceptance Skills.** There is an additional, specialized set of handouts and worksheets for **Skills When the Crisis Is Addiction.** One introductory handout precedes the handouts and worksheets on these skill sets:

• **Distress Tolerance Handout 1: Goals of Distress Tolerance.** The goals of distress tolerance are (1) to survive crisis situations without making them worse, (2) to accept reality as it is in the moment, and (3) to become free.

Crisis Survival Skills

• **Distress Tolerance Handout 2: Overview: Crisis Survival Skills.** The goal of crisis survival skills is to get through crises without making things worse. Crisis situations are, by definition, short-term. Thus these skills are not to be used all the time.

• **Distress Tolerance Worksheets 1, 1a, 1b: Crisis Survival Skills.** These are three different versions of worksheets that can be used with Handout 2 and throughout this portion of the module. Each worksheet covers all of the crisis survival skills.

• **Distress Tolerance Handout 3: When to Use Crisis Survival Skills.** This handout defines what a crisis is, and explains when and when not to use these skills.

• **Distress Tolerance Handout 4: The STOP Skill.** The STOP skill can keep you from acting impulsively on your emotions in ways that make a difficult situation worse. The term STOP is a way to remember how to do the skill: Stop, Take a step back, Observe, and Proceed mindfully. Two different worksheets can be used to track practice of the STOP skill—**Distress Tolerance Worksheets 2** and **2a: Practicing the STOP Skill.** Worksheet 2 provides space for two practices during the week. Worksheet 2a gives space for tracking daily practice.

• **Distress Tolerance Handout 5: Pros and Cons.** Listing pros and cons allows you to compare the advantages and disadvantages of different options. This particular handout asks you to compare the pros and cons of acting on your emotional urges in a crisis situation and of resisting those urges. Figure out and write down your pros and cons when you are *not* in a crisis; then, when a crisis hits, pull out your pros and cons and review them. You can also use **Distress Tolerance Worksheets 3** and **3a: Pros and Cons of Acting on Crisis Urges.** Both worksheets ask for the same information, but they are set up differently. Some people find one format much easier to work with than the other, and vice versa. Whichever one you use, remember to fill out all four quadrants.

• **Distress Tolerance Handout 6: TIP Skills: Changing Your Body Chemistry.** Very high emotion can make it impossible to use most skills. The TIP skills are designed as a quick way to reduce high emotional arousal. The TIP skills are Temperature (cold water), Intense exercise, Paced breathing, and Paired muscle relaxation. (Note that there are two P skills, although there is only one P in TIP.) There are also handouts on individual TIP skills as listed below. **Distress Tolerance Worksheet 4: Changing Body Chemistry with TIP Skills** covers all the TIP skills and can be used to track your practice.

• **Distress Tolerance Handout 6a: Using Cold Water, Step by Step.** This handout goes over how to use cold water to reduce emotional arousal quickly.

• **Distress Tolerance Handout 6b: Paired Muscle Relaxation, Step by Step.** Paired muscle relaxation is the pairing of relaxing your muscles with breathing out. The idea is to practice combining the two enough so that relaxing when highly emotional becomes easier and sometimes even automatic as you breathe out. This handout describes in detail how to practice paired muscle relaxation. To track your practice of this skill, use **Distress Tolerance Worksheet 4a: Paired Muscle Relaxation.**

• **Distress Tolerance Handout 6c: Effective Rethinking and Paired Relaxation.** This is a method of combining rethinking what you are telling yourself with paired relaxation to bring down emotion rapidly in moments of high stress. To track your practice of this skill, you can use **Distress Tolerance Worksheet 4b: Effective Rethinking and Paired Relaxation.**

• **Distress Tolerance Handout 7: Distracting.** Distracting methods work by reducing your contact with whatever set off the distress or its most painful aspects. The methods are listed on this handout and can be remembered with the term "Wise Mind ACCEPTS." There are three different worksheets for tracking practice—**Distress Tolerance Worksheets 5, 5a, and 5b: Distracting with Wise Mind ACCEPTS.** Worksheet 5 provides space for two practices between sessions. Worksheet 5a provides space for practicing every ACCEPTS skill twice. Worksheet 5b gives space for multiple practices of each skill.

• **Distress Tolerance Handout 8: Self-Soothing.** Self-soothing means doing things that feel pleasant and comforting, and that provide relief from stress or pain. It is being gentle and mindfully kind to yourself. This handout lists a number of ways to self-soothe through each of your five senses. There are three different worksheets you can use to track your self-soothing practice—**Distress Tolerance Worksheets 6, 6a, and 6b: Self-Soothing.** Each worksheet increases the number of practices, from two practices between sessions (Worksheet 6) to practice of each skill twice between sessions (Worksheet 6a) to multiple daily practices (Worksheet 6b).

• **Distress Tolerance Handout 8a: Body Scan Meditation, Step by Step.** This handout gives instructions for body scan meditation as a special form of self-soothing. Practice of the body scan can be recorded on **Distress Tolerance Worksheet 6c: Body Scan Meditation, Step by Step.**

• **Distress Tolerance Handout 9: Improving the Moment.** This handout lists a number of different strategies that can be used to improve the quality of the present moment, making it easier to survive a crisis without making it worse. The term IMPROVE is a way to remember the strategies. Any of three worksheets—**Distress Tolerance Worksheets 7, 7a, and 7b: IMPROVE the Moment**—can be used to track practice of this skill. Each worksheet increases the number of practices that can be recorded, from two practices during the week (Worksheet 7) to practice of every skill twice (Worksheet 7a) to multiple daily practices (Worksheet 7b).

• **Distress Tolerance Handout 9a: Sensory Awareness, Step by Step.** The R in IMPROVE stands for Relaxing actions, and sensory awareness is a relaxing action you can take to improve the moment. This handout can be used as a guide to this exercise.

Reality Acceptance Skills

• **Distress Tolerance Handout 10: Overview: Reality Acceptance Skills.** The goal of reality acceptance is to reduce suffering and increase a sense of freedom by finding ways to accept the facts of your life. This handout briefly lists the six reality acceptance skills.

• **Distress Tolerance Worksheets 8, 8a, 8b: Reality Acceptance Skills.** These three worksheets cover practice of all the reality acceptance skills. They can be used to track practice of any of the skills in this section. There are also worksheets for specific reality acceptance skills, as mentioned below.

• **Distress Tolerance Handout 11: Radical Acceptance.** Radical acceptance is a complete and total openness to the facts of reality as they are, without fighting the facts or being willful and ineffective. This handout outlines what has to be accepted and why radical acceptance is better than nonacceptance. It is helpful to use this handout with **Distress Tolerance Worksheet 9: Radical Acceptance** which helps you figure out what you might need to radically accept.

• **Distress Tolerance Handout 11a: Radical Acceptance: Factors That Interfere.** This handout clarifies what radical acceptance is not and outlines factors that interfere with it.

• **Distress Tolerance Handout 11b: Practicing Radical Acceptance, Step by Step.** This handout gives instructions for practicing radical acceptance. Practice can be recorded on Distress Tolerance Worksheet 9 as mentioned above, or on **Distress Tolerance Worksheet 9a: Practicing Radical Acceptance.**

• **Distress Tolerance Handout 12: Turning the Mind.** In order to accept reality that feels unacceptable, you usually have to make an effort more than once. You sometimes have to keep choosing to accept reality over and over for a very long time. Turning the mind is choosing to accept. This handout explains turning the mind and how to do it. Practice of this skill can be tracked on **Distress Tolerance Worksheet 10: Turning the Mind, Willingness, Willfulness.**

• **Distress Tolerance Handout 13: Willingness.** Willingness is the readiness to respond to life's situations wisely, as needed, voluntarily, and without grudge. It is the opposite of willfulness. This handout describes how to practice willingness. As with Handout 12, practice can be recorded on Distress Tolerance Worksheet 10.

• **Distress Tolerance Handout 14: Half-Smiling and Willing Hands.** Half smiling and willing hands are two ways to accept reality with your body. This handout describes how to practice each skill. **Distress Tolerance Handout 14a: Practicing Half-Smiling and Willing Hands** describes several specific ways to practice these skills. Practice of these skills can be tracked on either **Distress Tolerance Worksheet 11: Half-Smiling and Willing Hands** or **11a: Practicing Half-Smiling and Willing Hands.** The two worksheets are similar, but Worksheet 11 requires more writing.

• **Distress Tolerance Handout 15: Mindfulness of Current Thoughts.** Mindfulness of current thoughts is observing thoughts as thoughts, as sensations of the brain, rather than as facts about the world. You simply let thoughts come and go—noticing them, but not trying to control or change them. Observing thoughts is similar to observing any other behavior. Handout 15 describes this skill. **Distress Tolerance Handout 15a: Practicing Mindfulness of Thoughts** lists examples of how to practice this skill. To record practice, you can use either of two worksheets—Distress Tolerance Worksheet 12: Mindfulness of Current Thoughts or Distress Tolerance Worksheet 12a: Practicing Mindfulness of Thoughts.

Skills When the Crisis Is Addiction

• **Distress Tolerance Handout 16: Overview: When the Crisis Is Addiction.** The skills in this special part of the module are specifically designed for dealing with various addictions. This handout lists these skills. **Distress Tolerance Worksheet 13: Skills When the Crisis Is Addiction** covers all these skills and can be used instead of worksheets for the specific skills mentioned below.

- **Distress Tolerance Handout 16a: Common Addictions.** This handout defines addiction and lists common behaviors that can become addictions when you are unable to stop them, despite your best efforts to stop and despite negative consequences.

- **Distress Tolerance Handout 17: Dialectical Abstinence.** Dialectical abstinence is the synthesis of absolute abstinence (total commitment to abstinence) and harm reduction (planning for slips into the addictive behavior so they don't become relapses).

- **Distress Tolerance Handout 17a: Planning for Dialectical Abstinence.** This handout lists ways to plan for both abstinence and harm reduction. The items under "Plan for Abstinence" are shorthand for the skills described on Distress Tolerance Handouts 18–21. To track your practice of dialectical abstinence, use **Distress Tolerance Worksheet 14: Planning for Dialectical Abstinence.**

- **Distress Tolerance Handout 18: Clear Mind.** "Clear mind" is the middle ground between the extremes of "addict mind" (when you are governed by your addiction) and "clean mind" (when you think your problems are behind you and you don't need to be careful of a potential relapse). Clear mind is the safest place to be, since it involves not engaging in the addictive behavior while remaining vigilant of the temptation to do so.

- **Distress Tolerance Handout 18a: Behavior Patterns Characteristic of Addict Mind and of Clean Mind.** This handout lists typical behaviors of addict mind and clean mind and can help you identify when you are in one or the other. In particular, check the behaviors you engage in while you are in clean mind. Use **Distress Tolerance Worksheet 15: From Clean Mind to Clear Mind** to practice replacing clean mind behaviors you've marked on Handout 18a with clear mind behaviors.

- **Distress Tolerance Handout 19: Community Reinforcement.** Community reinforcement means restructuring your environment so that it will reinforce abstinence instead of addiction. This handout explains why this is important and lists steps you can take to make it happen. Use **Distress Tolerance Worksheet 16: Reinforcing Nonaddictive Behaviors** to track your practice of community reinforcement.

- **Distress Tolerance Handout 20: Burning Bridges and Building New Ones.** "Burning bridges" here means actively eliminating from your life any and every connection to potential triggers for addictive behaviors. "Building new bridges" means creating new visual images and smells in your mind to compete with addiction urges. Use **Distress Tolerance Worksheet 17: Burning Bridges and Building New Ones** to track your practice of this skill.

- **Distress Tolerance Handout 21: Alternate Rebellion and Adaptive Denial.** When addiction functions as rebellion, you can use some type of alternate rebellion to satisfy your wish to rebel without destroying yourself or blocking your way to achieving important goals. Adaptive denial consists of convincing yourself that you actually don't crave the addictive behavior (denial). The first half of this handout lists possible forms of alternate rebellion. The second half of the handout describes steps for adaptive denial. Use **Distress Tolerance Worksheet 18: Practicing Alternate Rebellion and Adaptive Denial** to track your practice of these skills.

Distress Tolerance Handouts

Goals of Distress Tolerance

SURVIVE CRISIS SITUATIONS

Without Making Them Worse

ACCEPT REALITY

**Replace Suffering and Being "Stuck"
with Ordinary Pain and the Possibility of Moving Forward**

BECOME FREE

**Of Having to Satisfy
the Demands of Your Own
Desires, Urges, and Intense Emotions**

OTHER: _____

Handouts for Crisis Survival Skills

Overview:
Crisis Survival Skills

These are skills for tolerating painful events, urges, and emotions when you cannot make things better right away.

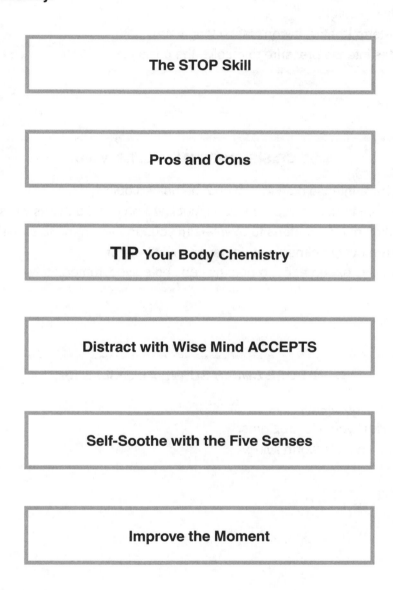

The STOP Skill

Pros and Cons

TIP Your Body Chemistry

Distract with Wise Mind ACCEPTS

Self-Soothe with the Five Senses

Improve the Moment

When to Use Crisis Survival Skills

YOU ARE IN A CRISIS when the situation is:

- Highly stressful.
- Short-term (that is, it won't last a long time).
- Creates intense pressure to resolve the crisis *now*.

USE CRISIS SURVIVAL SKILLS when:

1. You have intense pain that cannot be helped quickly.
2. You want to act on your emotions, but it will only make things worse.
3. Emotion mind threatens to overwhelm you, and you need to stay skillful.
4. You are overwhelmed, yet demands must be met.
5. Arousal is extreme, but problems can't be solved immediately.

DON'T USE CRISIS SURVIVAL SKILLS for:

- Everyday problems.
- Solving all your life problems.
- Making your life worth living.

STOP Skill

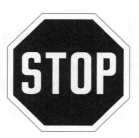

Stop — Do not just react. Stop! Freeze! Do not move a muscle! Your emotions may try to make you act without thinking. Stay in control!

Take a step back — Take a step back from the situation. Take a break. Let go. Take a deep breath. Do not let your feelings make you act impulsively.

Observe — Notice what is going on inside and outside you. What is the situation? What are your thoughts and feelings? What are others saying or doing?

Proceed mindfully — Act with awareness. In deciding what to do, consider your thoughts and feelings, the situation, and other people's thoughts and feelings. Think about your goals. Ask Wise Mind: Which actions will make it better or worse?

Note. Adapted from an unpublished worksheet by Francheska Perepletchikova and Seth Axelrod, with their permission.

Pros and Cons

Use pros and cons any time you have to decide between two courses of action.

❑ An urge is a crisis when it is very strong and when acting on the urge will make things *worse* in the long term.

❑ Make a list of the pros *and* cons of acting on your crisis urges. These might be to engage in dangerous, addictive, or harmful behaviors, or they might be to give in, give up, or avoid doing what is necessary to build a life you want to live.

❑ Make another list of the pros and cons of resisting crisis urges—that is, tolerating the distress and not giving in to the urges.

❑ Use the grid below to evaluate both sets of pros and cons (this type of grid is also used in Distress Tolerance Worksheet 3). Or you can use the type of grid seen in Distress Tolerance Worksheet 3a and in the pros-and-cons worksheets for other modules.

	PROS	**CONS**
Acting on crisis urges	**Pros** of acting on impulsive urges, giving in, giving up, or avoiding what needs to be done. _____ _____ _____ _____	**Cons** of acting on impulsive urges, giving in, giving up, or avoiding what needs to be done. _____ _____ _____ _____
Resisting crisis urges	**Pros** of resisting impulsive urges, doing what needs to be done, and not giving up. _____ _____ _____ _____	**Cons** of resisting impulsive urges, doing what needs to be done, and not giving up. _____ _____ _____ _____

Before an overwhelming crisis urge hits:

Write out your pros and cons; carry them with you.
Rehearse your pros and cons over and over.

When an overwhelming crisis urge hits:

Review your pros and cons. Get out your list and read it over again.

- Imagine the positive consequences of resisting the urge.
- Think of the negative consequences of giving in to crisis behaviors.
- Remember past consequences when you have acted on crisis urges.

TIP Skills: Changing Your Body Chemistry

To reduce extreme emotion mind *fast*.

Remember these as **TIP** skills:

T

> ### <u>T</u>IP THE <u>T</u>EMPERATURE of your face with COLD WATER*
> ### (to calm down fast)
>
> - Holding your breath, put your face in a bowl of cold water,
>   or hold a cold pack (or zip-lock bag of cold water) on your eyes and cheeks.
> - Hold for 30 seconds. Keep water above 50°F.

I

> ### <u>I</u>NTENSE EXERCISE*
> ### (to calm down your body when it is revved up by emotion)
>
> - Engage in intense exercise, if only for a short while.
>
> - Expend your body's stored up physical energy by running, walking fast, jumping,
>   playing basketball, lifting weights, etc.

P

> ### <u>P</u>ACED BREATHING
> ### (pace your breathing by slowing it down)
>
> - Breathe deeply into your belly.
> - Slow your pace of inhaling and exhaling way down (on average, five to six breaths
>   per minute).
> - Breathe *out* more slowly than you breathe *in* (for example, 5 seconds in and 7
>   seconds out).

> ### <u>P</u>AIRED MUSCLE RELAXATION
> ### (to calm down by pairing muscle relaxation with breathing out)
>
> - While breathing into your belly deeply tense your body muscles (*not* so much as
>   to cause a cramp).
> - Notice the tension in your body.
> - While breathing out, say the word "Relax" in your mind.
> - Let go of the tension.
> - Notice the difference in your body.

*Caution: Very cold water decreases your heart rate rapidly. Intense exercise will increase heart rate. Consult your health care provider before using these skills if you have a heart or medical condition, a lowered base heart rate due to medications, take a beta-blocker, are allergic to cold, or have an eating disorder.

Using Cold Water, Step by Step

COLD WATER CAN WORK WONDERS*

When you put your full face into cold water . . . **or** you put a zip-lock bag with cold water on your eyes and upper cheeks, and **hold your breath,** it tells your brain you are diving underwater.

This causes the **"dive response"** to occur. (It may take 15–30 seconds to start.)

Your heart slows down, blood flow to nonessential organs is reduced, and blood flow is redirected to the brain and heart.

This response can actually help **regulate your emotions.**

This will be useful as a **distress tolerance strategy** when you are having a very **strong, distressing emotion,** or when you are having very **strong urges to engage in dangerous behaviors**.

(This strategy works best when you are sitting quietly—activity and distraction may make it less effective.)

TRY IT OUT!

Caution: Very cold water decreases your heart rate. If you have any heart or medical condition, have a lowered base heart rate due to medications, or are on a beta-blocker, consult your health care provider before using these skills. Avoid ice water if you are allergic to the cold.

Paired Muscle Relaxation, Step by Step

If you have decided to practice **paired muscle relaxation,** it can be very helpful to practice relaxing each of your muscles first.

When you are starting, practice in a quiet place to reduce distractions, and make sure that you have enough time. As you improve with practice, you will want to practice in many different kinds of places, so that you can relax effectively when you most need to.

Remember that effectiveness improves with practice. If judgments arise, observe them, let them go, and return to your practice. If you become anxious, try focusing on breathing *in* to the count of 5 and *out* to the count of 7 (or the counts you have already determined for paced breathing), breathing all the while into your belly until you can return to relaxation exercises.

Now that you are ready to begin . . .

1. Get your body into a comfortable position in which you can relax. Loosen tight clothing. Lie or sit down, with all body parts uncrossed and no body part supporting any others.
2. For each area of the body listed below, gather tension by tightening muscles. Focus on the sensation of tightness in and around that area. Hold the tension as you inhale for 5–6 seconds, then release and breathe out.
3. As you release, say in your mind very slowly the word "Relax."
4. Observe the changes in sensations as you relax for 10–15 seconds then move on to the next muscle.

> Start first with each of the 16 muscle groups.
> Once you can do that, practice with medium groups of muscles and then large groups.
> Once you are good at that, practice tensing your entire body at once.
>
> When you tense your entire body, you are like a robot—stiff, nothing moving.
> When you relax your entire body, you are like a rag doll—all muscles drooping down.
>
> Once you can relax all your muscles, practice three or four times a day until you can routinely relax your entire body rapidly.
> By practicing pairing exhaling and the word "Relax" with relaxing your muscles, you will eventually be able to relax just by letting go and saying the word "Relax."

Large Medium Small

1. Hands and wrists: Make fists with both hands and pull fists up on the wrists.
2. Lower and upper arms: Make fists and bend both arms up to touch your shoulders.
3. Shoulders: Pull both shoulders up to your ears.
4. Forehead: Pull eyebrows close together, wrinkling forehead.
5. Eyes: Shut eyes tightly.
6. Nose and upper cheeks: Scrunch up nose; bring upper lips and cheeks up toward eyes.
7. Lips and lower face: Press lips together; bring edges of lips back toward ears.
8. Tongue and mouth: Teeth together; tongue pushing on upper mouth.
9. Neck: Push head back into chair, floor, or bed, or push chin down to chest.
10. Chest: Take deep breath and hold it.
11. Back: Arch back, bringing shoulder blades together.
12. Stomach: Hold stomach in tightly.
13. Buttocks: Squeeze buttocks together.
14. Upper legs and thighs: Legs out; tense thighs.
15. Calves: Legs out; point toes down.
16. Ankles: Legs out; point toes together, heels out, toes curled under.

Remember, paired relaxation is a skill. It takes time to develop. With practice, you will notice the benefits.

Note. Adapted from Smith, R. E. (1980). Development of an integrated coping response through cognitive–affective stress management training. In I. G. Sarason & C. D. Spielberger (Eds.), *Stress and anxiety* (Vol. 7, pp. 265–280). Washington, DC: Hemisphere. Copyright 1980 by Hemisphere Publishing Corporation. Adapted by permission.

Effective Rethinking and Paired Relaxation, Step by Step

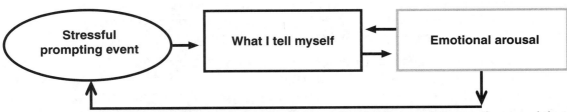

Step 1. Write down the **prompting event** that is often related to distressing emotions and that you want to work on reducing your emotional reactions to.

Step 2. Ask: "What must I be telling myself (that is, what are my **interpretations and thoughts**) about the event that causes such distress and arousal?" Write these down. Examples:

"He hates me," "I can't stand this!" "I can't do this," "I'll never make it," "I'm out of control!"

Step 3. Rethink the situation and its meaning in a way that counteracts the thoughts and interpretations producing stress and distressing emotions. As you rethink the situation, write down as many **effective thoughts** as you can to replace the stressful thoughts.

Step 4. When you are *not* in the stressful prompting event, **practice imagining** the stressful event:

   a. At the same time, while **breathing in,** say to yourself an effective self-statement.
   b. When **breathing out, say** "Relax" while intentionally relaxing all your muscles.

Step 5. Keep practicing every chance you get until you have mastered the strategy.

Step 6. When a stressful situation occurs, practice effective rethinking and paired relaxation.

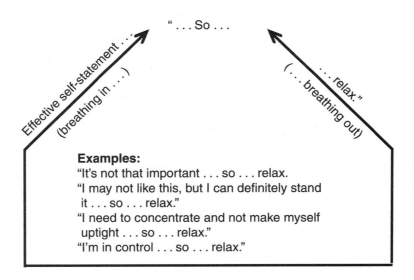

Examples:
"It's not that important . . . so . . . relax.
"I may not like this, but I can definitely stand it . . . so . . . relax."
"I need to concentrate and not make myself uptight . . . so . . . relax."
"I'm in control . . . so . . . relax."

Note. Adapted from Smith, R. E. (1980). Development of an integrated coping response through cognitive–affective stress management training. In I. G. Sarason & C. D. Spielberger (Eds.), *Stress and anxiety* (Vol. 7, pp. 265–280). Washington, DC: Hemisphere. Copyright 1980 by Hemisphere Publishing Corporation. Adapted by permission.

Distracting

A way to remember these skills is the phrase **"Wise Mind ACCEPTS."**

With **Activities:**

❑ Focus attention on a task you need to get done.
❑ Rent movies; watch TV.
❑ Clean a room in your house.
❑ Find an event to go to.
❑ Play computer games.
❑ Go walking. Exercise.
❑ Surf the Internet. Write e-mails.
❑ Play sports.

❑ Go out for a meal or eat a favorite food.
❑ Call or go out with a friend.
❑ Listen to your iPod; download music.
❑ Build something.
❑ Spend time with your children.
❑ Play cards.
❑ Read magazines, books, comics.
❑ Do crossword puzzles or Sudoku.
❑ Other: _____

With **Contributing:**

❑ Find volunteer work to do.
❑ Help a friend or family member.
❑ Surprise someone with something nice (a card, a favor, a hug).
❑ Give away things you don't need.

❑ Call or send an instant message encouraging someone or just saying hi.
❑ Make something nice for someone else.
❑ Do something thoughtful.
❑ Other: _____

With **Comparisons:**

❑ Compare how you are feeling now to a time when you felt different.
❑ Think about people coping the same as you or less well than you.

❑ Compare yourself to those less fortunate.
❑ Watch reality shows about others' troubles; read about disasters, others' suffering.
❑ Other: _____

With different **Emotions:**

❑ Read emotional books or stories, old letters.
❑ Watch emotional TV shows; go to emotional movies.
❑ Listen to emotional music.
(Be sure the event creates different emotions.)

Ideas: Scary movies, joke books, comedies, funny records, religious music, soothing music or music that fires you up, going to a store and reading funny greeting cards.
❑ Other: _____

With **Pushing away:**

❑ Push the situation away by leaving it for a while.
❑ Leave the situation mentally.
❑ Build an imaginary wall between yourself and the situation.
❑ Block thoughts and images from your mind.

❑ Notice ruminating: Yell "No!"
❑ Refuse to think about the painful situations.
❑ Put the pain on a shelf. Box it up and put it away for a while.
❑ Deny the problem for the moment.
❑ Other: _____

With other **Thoughts:**

❑ Count to 10; count colors in a painting or poster or out the window; count anything.
❑ Repeat words to a song in your mind.

❑ Work puzzles.
❑ Watch TV or read.
❑ Other: _____

With other **Sensations:**

❑ Squeeze a rubber ball very hard.
❑ Listen to very loud music.
❑ Hold ice in your hand or mouth.

❑ Go out in the rain or snow.
❑ Take a hot or cold shower.
❑ Other: _____

Self-Soothing

A way to remember these skills is to think of soothing each of your **FIVE SENSES.**

With **Vision:**

- ☐ Look at the stars at night.
- ☐ Look at pictures you like in a book.
- ☐ Buy one beautiful flower.
- ☐ Make one space in a room pleasing to look at.
- ☐ Light a candle and watch the flame.
- ☐ Set a pretty place at the table using your best things.
- ☐ Go people-watching or window-shopping.
- ☐ Go to a museum or poster shop with beautiful art.
- ☐ Sit in the lobby of a beautiful old hotel.
- ☐ Look at nature around you.
- ☐ Walk in a pretty part of town.
- ☐ Watch a sunrise or a sunset.
- ☐ Go to a dance performance, or watch it on TV.
- ☐ Be mindful of each sight that passes in front of you.
- ☐ Take a walk in a park or a scenic hike.
- ☐ Browse through stores looking at things.
- ☐ Other: _____

With **Hearing:**

- ☐ Listen to soothing or invigorating music.
- ☐ Pay attention to sounds of nature (waves, birds, rainfall, leaves rustling).
- ☐ Pay attention to the sounds of the city (traffic, horns, city music).
- ☐ Sing to your favorite songs.
- ☐ Hum a soothing tune.
- ☐ Learn to play an instrument.
- ☐ Burn a CD or make an iPod mix with music that will get you through tough times. Turn it on.
- ☐ Be mindful of any sounds that come your way, letting them go in one ear and out the other.
- ☐ Turn on the radio.
- ☐ Other: _____

With **Smell:**

- ☐ Use your favorite soap, shampoo, aftershave, cologne, or lotions, or try them on in the store.
- ☐ Burn incense or light a scented candle.
- ☐ Open a package of coffee and inhale the aroma.
- ☐ Put lemon oil on your furniture.
- ☐ Put potpourri or eucalyptus oil in a bowl in your room.
- ☐ Sit in a new car and breathe the aroma.
- ☐ Boil cinnamon. Make cookies, bread, or popcorn.
- ☐ Smell the roses.
- ☐ Walk in a wooded area and mindfully breathe in the fresh smells of nature.
- ☐ Open the window and smell the air.
- ☐ Other: _____

With **Taste:**

- ☐ Eat some of your favorite foods.
- ☐ Drink your favorite soothing drink, such as herbal tea, hot chocolate, a latté, or a smoothie.
- ☐ Treat yourself to a dessert.
- ☐ Eat macaroni and cheese or another favorite childhood food.
- ☐ Sample flavors in an ice cream store.
- ☐ Suck on a piece of peppermint candy.
- ☐ Chew your favorite gum.
- ☐ Get a little bit of a special food you don't usually spend the money on, such as fresh-squeezed orange juice or your favorite candy.
- ☐ Really taste the food you eat. Eat one thing mindfully.
- ☐ Other: _____

With **Touch:**

- ☐ Take a long hot bath or shower.
- ☐ Pet your dog or cat.
- ☐ Have a massage. Soak your feet.
- ☐ Put creamy lotion on your whole body.
- ☐ Put a cold compress on your forehead.
- ☐ Sink into a comfortable chair in your home.
- ☐ Put on a blouse or shirt that has a pleasant feel.
- ☐ Take a drive with the car windows rolled down.
- ☐ Run your hand along smooth wood or leather.
- ☐ Hug someone.
- ☐ Put clean sheets on the bed.
- ☐ Wrap up in a blanket.
- ☐ Notice touch that is soothing.
- ☐ Other: _____

Body Scan Meditation Step by Step

Sit on a chair, or lie on your back on the floor with legs uncrossed. Put your arms in a comfortable position by your side, on your abdomen, or (if sitting) put them on your thighs palms up. Open your eyes partially to let light in. If you are lying on the floor, put a cushion under your knees if need be. Imagine your breath flowing to each part of your body as your attention gently moves up your body. Adopt a mind of curiosity and interest as you focus on each part of your body.

Focus on your breathing. Notice how the air moves in and out of your body.

- Take several deep breaths until you begin to feel comfortable and relaxed.
- Direct your attention to the *toes* of your left foot.
- Notice the sensations in that part of your body while remaining aware of your breathing.
- Imagine each breath flowing to your *toes*.
- Looking with curiosity, ask, "What am I feeling in this part of my body?"
- Focus on your left *toes* for several minutes.

- Then move your focus to the *arch* and *heel* of your left foot, and hold it there for a minute or two while continuing to pay attention to your breathing.
- Notice the sensations on your skin of warmth or coldness; notice the weight of your foot on the floor.
- Imagine your breath flowing to the *arch* and *heel* of your left foot.
- Ask, "What are the feelings in the *arch* and *heel* of my left foot?"

- Follow the same procedure as you move to your left *ankle*, *calf*, *knee*, *upper legs*, and *thigh*.
- Repeat with the right leg, starting with your toes.
- Then move through your *pelvis*, and *lower back*, and around to your *stomach*.
- Focus on the rising and falling of your belly as your breath goes in and out.
- Then go on to your *chest*; *left hand*, *arm*, and *shoulder*; *right hand*, *arm*, and *shoulder*; *neck*, *chin*, *tongue*, *mouth*, *lips*, and *lower face*; and *nose*.
- Notice your breath as it comes in and out of your nostrils.
- Then focus on your upper cheeks, eyes, forehead, and scalp.

- Finally, focus on the very top of your hair.
- Then let go of your body altogether.

Don't worry if you notice that thoughts, sounds, or other sensations come into your awareness. Just notice them and then gently refocus your mind. Don't worry if your mind has been drawn away from the object of your attention and you find yourself thinking about something else (it nearly always happens). Just calmly, gently, but with resolution, turn your mind back to the part of the body you've reached. You may need to bring your attention back over and over. You are not alone in this. It is this bringing of your attention back over and over and over, without judgment or harshness, that is the essential element of the meditation.

Improving the Moment

A way to remember these skills is the word **IMPROVE.**

With **Imagery:**

❑ Imagine very relaxing scenes.
❑ Imagine a secret room within yourself. Furnish it the way you like. Close and lock the door on anything that can hurt you.
❑ Imagine everything going well.
❑ Make up a calming fantasy world.

❑ Imagine hurtful emotions draining out of you like water out of a pipe.
❑ Remember a happy time and imagine yourself in it again; play out the time in your mind again.
❑ Other: _____

With **Meaning:**

❑ Find purpose or meaning in a painful situation.
❑ Focus on whatever positive aspects of a painful situation you can find.
❑ Repeat these positive aspects in your mind.

❑ Remember, listen to, or read about spiritual values.
❑ Other: _____

With **Prayer:**

❑ Open your heart to a supreme being, God, or your own Wise Mind.
❑ Ask for strength to bear the pain.

❑ Turn things over to God or a higher being.
❑ Other: _____

With **Relaxing** actions:

❑ Take a hot bath or sit in a hot tub.
❑ Drink hot milk.
❑ Massage your neck and scalp.
❑ Practice yoga or other stretching.

❑ Breathe deeply.
❑ Change your facial expression.
❑ Other: _____

With **One thing in the moment:**

❑ Focus your entire attention on just what you are doing.
❑ Keep yourself in the moment.
❑ Put your mind in the present.

❑ Focus your entire attention on the physical
❑ Listen to a sensory awareness recording (or use Distress Tolerance Handout 9a)
❑ Other: _____

With a brief **Vacation:**

❑ Give yourself a brief vacation.
❑ Get in bed; pull the covers up over your head.
❑ Go to the beach or the woods for the day.
❑ Get a magazine and read it with chocolates.
❑ Turn off your phone for a day.

❑ Take a blanket to the park and sit on it for a whole afternoon.
❑ Take a 1-hour breather from hard work.
❑ Take a brief vacation from responsibility.
❑ Other: _____

With self-**Encouragement and rethinking the situation:**

❑ Cheerlead yourself: "You go, girl!" "You da man!"
❑ "I will make it out of this."
❑ "I'm doing the best I can."
❑ Repeat over and over: "I can stand it."

❑ "This too shall pass."
❑ "I will be OK."
❑ "It won't last forever."
❑ Other: _____

List (and then practice) rethoughts that are particularly important in your crisis situations (e.g., "The fact that he did not pick me up doesn't mean he doesn't love me"):
❑ _____   ❑ _____

Sensory Awareness, Step by Step

Find a comfortable position. Staying in this position, listen to the questions below, listening for your response after each question. If you do not have a recording of these questions, you can make one for yourself (or ask a friend to make one), recording each question with about 5 seconds between each question.

1. Can you feel your hair touching your head?
2. Can you feel your belly rising and falling as you breathe?
3. Can you feel the space between your eyes?
4. Can you feel the distance between your ears?
5. Can you feel your breath touching the back of your eyes while you inhale?
6. Can you picture something far away?
7. Can you notice your arms touching your body?
8. Can you feel the bottoms of your feet?
9. Can you imagine a beautiful day at the beach?
10. Can you notice the space within your mouth?
11. Can you notice the position of your tongue in your mouth?
12. Can you feel a breeze against your cheek?
13. Can you feel how one arm is heavier than the other?
14. Can you feel a tingling or numbness in one hand?
15. Can you feel how one arm is more relaxed than the other?
16. Can you feel a change in the temperature in the air around you?
17. Can you feel how your left arm is warmer than the right?
18. Can you imagine how it would feel to be a rag doll?
19. Can you notice any tightness in your left forearm?
20. Can you imagine something very pleasant?
21. Can you imagine what it would feel like to float on a cloud?
22. Can you imagine what it would feel like to be stuck in molasses?
23. Can you picture something far away?
24. Can you feel a heaviness in your legs?
25. Can you imagine floating in warm water?
26. Can you notice your body hanging on your bones?
27. Can you allow yourself to drift lazily?
28. Can you feel your face getting soft?
29. Can you imagine a beautiful flower?
30. Can you feel how one arm and leg are heavier than the other?

Note. Items 29 and 30 are adapted from Goldfried, M. R., & Davison, G. C. (1976). *Clinical behavior therapy.* New York: Holt, Rinehart & Winston. Copyright 1976 by Marvin R. Goldfried and Gerald C. Davison. Adapted by permission of the authors.

Handouts for Reality Acceptance Skills

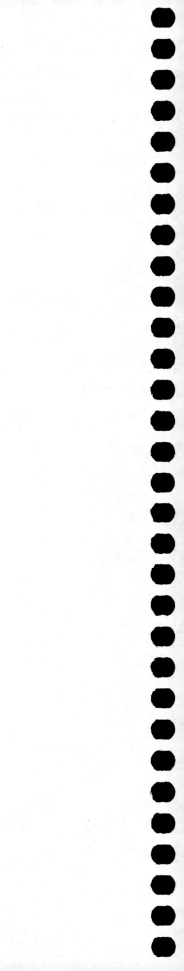

Overview:
Reality Acceptance Skills

These are skills for how to live a life that is not the life you want.

RADICAL ACCEPTANCE

TURNING THE MIND

WILLINGNESS

HALF-SMILING AND WILLING HANDS

ALLOWING THE MIND: MINDFULNESS OF CURRENT THOUGHTS

Radical Acceptance

(When you cannot keep painful events and emotions from coming your way.)

WHAT IS RADICAL ACCEPTANCE?

1. Radical means *all the way*, complete and total.

2. It is accepting in your mind, your heart, and your body.

3. It's when you stop fighting reality, stop throwing tantrums because reality is not the way you want it, and let go of bitterness.

WHAT HAS TO BE ACCEPTED?

1. Reality is as it is (the facts about the past and the present are the facts, even if you don't like them).

2. There are limitations on the future for everyone (but only realistic limitations need to be accepted).

3. Everything has a cause (including events and situations that cause you pain and suffering).

4. Life can be worth living even with painful events in it.

WHY ACCEPT REALITY?

1. Rejecting reality does not change reality.

2. Changing reality requires first accepting reality.

3. Pain can't be avoided; it is nature's way of signaling that something is wrong.

4. Rejecting reality turns pain into suffering.

5. Refusing to accept reality can keep you stuck in unhappiness, bitterness, anger, sadness, shame, or other painful emotions.

6. Acceptance may lead to sadness, but deep calmness usually follows.

7. The path out of hell is through misery. By refusing to accept the misery that is part of climbing out of hell, you fall back into hell.

Radical Acceptance: Factors That Interfere

RADICAL ACCEPTANCE IS <u>NOT</u>:

Approval, compassion, love, passivity, or against change.

FACTORS THAT INTERFERE WITH ACCEPTANCE

❏ 1. You don't have the skills for acceptance; you do not know how to accept really painful events and facts.

❏ 2. You believe that if you accept a painful event, you are making light of it or are approving of the facts, and that nothing will be done to change or prevent future painful events.

❏ 3. Emotions get in the way (unbearable sadness; anger at the person or group that caused the painful event; rage at the injustice of the world; overwhelming shame about who you are; guilt about your own behavior).

❏ Other: _____

Practicing Radical Acceptance Step by Step

❑ Observe that you are questioning or fighting reality ("It shouldn't be this way").

❑ Remind yourself that the unpleasant reality is just as it is and cannot be changed ("This is what happened").

❑ Remind yourself that there are causes for the reality. Acknowledge that some sort of history led up to this very moment. Consider how people's lives have been shaped by a series of factors. Notice that given these causal factors and how history led up to this moment, this reality had to occur just this way ("This is how things happened").

❑ Practice accepting with the whole self (mind, body, and spirit). Be creative in finding ways to involve your whole self. Use accepting self-talk—but also consider using relaxation; mindfulness of your breath; half-smiling and willing hands while thinking about what feels unacceptable; prayer; going to a place that helps bring you to acceptance; or imagery.

❑ Practice opposite action. List all the behaviors you would do if you did accept the facts. Then act as if you have already accepted the facts. Engage in the behaviors that you would do if you really had accepted.

❑ Cope ahead with events that seem unacceptable. Imagine (in your mind's eye) believing what you don't want to accept. Rehearse in your mind what you would do if you accepted what seems unacceptable.

❑ Attend to body sensations as you think about what you need to accept.

❑ Allow disappointment, sadness, or grief to arise within you.

❑ Acknowledge that life can be worth living even when there is pain.

❑ Do pros and cons if you find yourself resisting practicing acceptance.

Turning the Mind

TURNING THE MIND is like facing a fork in the road. You have to turn your mind toward the acceptance road, and away from the road of rejecting reality.

TURNING THE MIND is choosing to accept.

The CHOICE to accept does not itself equal acceptance. It just puts you on the path.

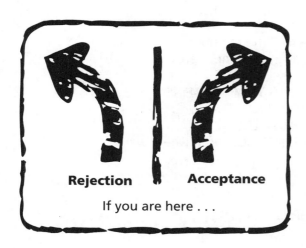

Rejection   **Acceptance**

If you are here . . .

TURNING THE MIND, STEP BY STEP

1. **OBSERVE** that you are not accepting. (Look for anger, bitterness, annoyance; avoiding emotions; saying "Why me?", "Why is this happening?", "I can't stand this," "It shouldn't be this way.")

2. Go within yourself and **MAKE AN INNER COMMITMENT** to accept reality as it is.

3. **DO IT AGAIN,** over and over. Keep turning your mind to acceptance each time you come to the fork in the road where you can reject reality or accept it.

4. **DEVELOP A PLAN** for catching yourself in the future when you drift out of acceptance.

Willingness

Willingness is readiness to enter and participate fully in life and living.

Find a WILLING RESPONSE to each situation.

Willingness is DOING JUST WHAT IS NEEDED:

- In each situation.
- Wholeheartedly, without dragging your feet.

Willingness is listening very carefully to your WISE MIND, and then acting from your WISE MIND.

Willingness is ACTING WITH AWARENESS that you are connected to the universe (to the stars, people you like and don't like, the floor, etc.).

Replace WILLFULNESS with WILLINGNESS.

- Willfulness is **REFUSING TO TOLERATE** the moment.
- Willfulness is refusing to make changes that are needed.
- Willfulness is **GIVING UP.**
- Willfulness is the **OPPOSITE OF "DOING WHAT WORKS."**
- Willfulness is trying to **FIX EVERY SITUATION.**
- Willfulness is insisting on **BEING IN CONTROL.**
- Willfulness is **ATTACHMENT TO "ME, ME, ME"** and "what I want right now!"

WILLINGNESS, STEP BY STEP

1. **OBSERVE** the willfulness. Label it. Experience it.
2. **RADICALLY ACCEPT** that at this moment you feel (and may be acting) willful. You cannot fight willfulness with willfulness.
3. **TURN YOUR MIND** toward acceptance and willingness.
4. **Try HALF-SMILING** and a **WILLING POSTURE.**
5. When willfulness is immovable, **ASK, "WHAT'S THE THREAT?"**

Situations where I notice my own:

Willfulness: _____

Willingness: _____

Half-Smiling and Willing Hands

Accepting reality with your body.

HALF-SMILING

1st. *Relax* your face from the top of your head down to your chin and jaw.

Let go of each facial muscle (forehead, eyes, and brows; cheeks, mouth, and tongue; teeth slightly apart). If you have difficulty, try tensing your facial muscles and then letting go.

A tense smile is a grin (and might tell your brain you are hiding or masking your real feelings).

2nd. Let both *corners of your lips* go slightly up, just so you can feel them.

It is not necessary for others to see it. A half-smile is slightly upturned lips with a relaxed face.

3rd. Try to adopt a serene facial expression.

Remember, your face communicates to your brain; your body connects to your mind.

WILLING HANDS

Standing: Drop your arms down from your shoulders; keep them straight or bent slightly at the elbows. With hands unclenched, turn your hands outward, with thumbs out to your sides, palms up, and fingers relaxed.

Sitting: Place your hands on your lap or your thighs. With hands unclenched, turn your hands outward, with palms up and fingers relaxed.

Lying down: Arms by your side, hands unclenched, turn your palms up with fingers relaxed.

Remember, your hands communicate to your brain; your body connects to your mind.

Practicing Half-Smiling and Willing Hands

1. **HALF-SMILE WHEN YOU FIRST WAKE UP IN THE MORNING.**

   Hang a branch, any other sign, or even the word "smile" on the ceiling or wall, so that you see it right away when you open your eyes. This sign will serve as your reminder. Use these seconds before you get out of bed to take hold of your breath. Inhale and exhale three breaths gently while maintaining a half-smile. Follow your breaths. Add willing hands to your half-smile, or practice willing hands alone.

2. **HALF-SMILE DURING YOUR FREE MOMENTS.**

   Anywhere you find yourself sitting or standing, half-smile. Look at a child, a leaf, a painting on a wall, or anything that is relatively still, and smile. Inhale and exhale quietly three times.

3. **HALF-SMILE WITH WILLING HANDS WHILE YOU ARE LISTENING TO MUSIC.**

   Listen to a piece of music for 2 or 3 minutes. Pay attention to the words, music, rhythm, and sentiments of the music you are listening to (not your daydreams of other times). Half-smile while watching your inhalations and exhalations. Adopt a willing-hands posture.

4. **HALF-SMILE WITH WILLING HANDS WHEN YOU ARE IRRITATED.**

   When you realize "I'm irritated," half-smile or adopt a willing-hands posture at once. Inhale and exhale quietly, maintaining a half-smile or willing hands for three breaths.

5. **HALF-SMILE IN A LYING-DOWN POSITION.**

   Lie on your back on a flat surface, without the support of mattress or pillow. Keep your two arms loosely by your sides, and keep your two legs slightly apart, stretched out before you. Maintain willing hands and a half-smile. Breathe in and out gently, keeping your attention focused on your breath. Let go of every muscle in your body. Relax each muscle as though it were sinking down through the floor, or as though it were as soft and yielding as a piece of silk hanging in the breeze to dry. Let go entirely, keeping your attention only on your breath and half-smile. Think of yourself as a cat, completely relaxed before a warm fire, whose muscles yield without resistance to anyone's touch. Continue for 15 breaths.

6. **HALF-SMILE IN A SITTING POSITION.**

   Sit on the floor with your back straight, or on a chair with your two feet touching the floor. Half-smile. Inhale and exhale while maintaining the half-smile. Let go.

(*continued on next page*)

Note. Exercises 1 and 3–7 are adapted from *The Miracle of Mindfulness* (pp. 77–81, 93) by Thich Nhat Hanh. Copyright 1975, 1976 by Thich Nhat Hanh. Preface and English translation copyright 1975, 1976, 1987 by Mobi Ho. Adapted by permission of Beacon Press, Boston.

7. HALF-SMILE WITH WILLING HANDS WHILE YOU ARE CONTEMPLATING A PERSON YOU DISLIKE OR ARE ANGRY WITH.

- Sit quietly. Breathe and smile a half-smile. Hold your hands open with palms up.

- Imagine the image of the person who has caused you suffering.

- Regard the features you dislike the most or find the most repulsive.

- Try to examine what makes this person happy and what causes suffering in his or her daily life.

- Imagine the person's perceptions; try to see what patterns of thought and reason this person follows.

- Examine what motivates this person's hopes and actions.

- Finally, consider the person's consciousness. See whether the person's views and insights are open and free or not, and whether or not the person has been influenced by any prejudices, narrow-mindedness, hatred, or anger.

- See whether or not the person is master of him- or herself.

- Continue until you feel compassion rise in your heart like a well filling with fresh water, and your anger and resentment disappear. Practice this exercise many times on the same person.

Notes/Other times to half-smile and/or form willing hands:

_____

_____

_____

_____

_____

_____

_____

_____

_____

_____

_____

_____

_____

_____

_____

Mindfulness of Current Thoughts

---

1. OBSERVE YOUR THOUGHTS.

- As waves, coming and going.
- Not suppressing thoughts.
- Not judging thoughts.
- Acknowledging their presence.
- Not keeping thoughts around.
- Not analyzing thoughts.
- Practicing willingness.
- Stepping back and observing thoughts as they run in and out of your mind.

---

2. ADOPT A CURIOUS MIND.

- Ask, "Where do my thoughts come from?" Watch and see.
- Notice that every thought that comes also goes out of your mind.
- Observe but do not evaluate your thoughts. Let go of judgments.

---

3. REMEMBER: YOU ARE NOT YOUR THOUGHTS.

- Do not necessarily act on thoughts.
- Remember times when you have had very different thoughts.
- Remind yourself that catastrophic thinking is "emotion mind."
- Remember how you think when you are not feeling such intense suffering and pain.

---

4. DON'T BLOCK OR SUPPRESS THOUGHTS.

- Ask, "What sensations are these thoughts trying to avoid?" Turn your mind to the sensation. Then come back to the thought. Repeat several times.
- Step back; allow your thoughts to come and go as you observe your breath.
- Play with your thoughts: Repeat them out loud over and over as fast as you can. Sing them. Imagine the thoughts as the words of a clown, as recordings getting all tangled up; as cute animals you can cuddle up to; as bright colors running through your mind; as only sounds.
- Try loving your thoughts.

Practicing Mindfulness of Thoughts

PRACTICE MINDFULNESS OF THOUGHTS BY OBSERVING THEM

☐ 1. Notice thoughts as they come into your mind. As a thought comes into your mind, say "a thought has entered my mind." Label the thought as a thought, saying, "The thought [describe thought] arose in my mind." Use a gentle voice tone.

☐ 2. As you notice thoughts in your mind, ask, "Where did the thought come from?" Then watch your mind to see if you can see where it came from.

☐ 3. Step back from your mind, as if you are on top of a mountain and your mind is just a boulder down below. Gaze at your mind, watching what thoughts come up when you are watching it. Come back into your mind before you stop.

☐ 4. Close your eyes and scan your body for the first physical sensation that you notice. Then scan your mind for the first thought you notice. Shuttle back and forth between scanning for physical sensations and scanning for thoughts. Another time, replace scanning your body for physical sensations to scanning yourself for any emotional feelings. Then shuttle back and forth between an emotional feeling and a thought.

PRACTICE MINDFULNESS OF THOUGHTS BY USING WORDS AND VOICE TONE

☐ 5. Verbalize thoughts or beliefs out loud, using a nonjudgmental voice tone, over and over and over:

    ☐ As fast as you can until the thoughts make no sense.

    ☐ Very, very slowly (one syllable or word per breath).

    ☐ In a different voice from yours (high- or low-pitched, like a cartoon character or celebrity).

    ☐ As a dialogue on a TV comedy show ("You'll never believe what thought went through my mind. I was thinking, 'I'm a jerk.' Can you believe that?").

    ☐ As songs, sung wholeheartedly and dramatically, in a tune that fits the thoughts.

PRACTICE MINDFULNESS OF THOUGHTS WITH OPPOSITE ACTION

☐ 6. Relax your face and body while imagining accepting your thoughts as only thoughts—sensations of the brain.

☐ 7. Imagine things you would do if you stopped believing everything you think.

☐ 8. Rehearse in your mind the things that you would do if you did not view your thoughts as facts.

☐ 9. Practice loving your thoughts as they go through your mind.

(*continued on next page*)

PRACTICE MINDFULNESS OF THOUGHTS BY IMAGINING THAT YOUR MIND IS:

❑ 10. A conveyor belt, and that thoughts and feelings are coming down the belt. Put each thought or feeling in a box labeled with the type of thought that it is (e.g., worry thoughts, thoughts about my past, thoughts about my mother, planning what to do thoughts). Just keep observing and sorting thoughts into the labeled boxes.

❑ 11. A river, and that thoughts and feelings are boats going down the river. Imagine sitting on the grass, watching the boats go by. Try not to jump on the boat.

❑ 12. A railroad track, and that thoughts and feelings are train cars going by. Try not to jump on the train.

❑ 13. A leaf that has dropped off a tree into a beautiful creek flowing by you as you sit on the grass. Each time a thought or image comes into your mind, imagine that it is written or pictured on the leaf floating by. Let each leaf go by, watching as it goes out of sight.

❑ 14. The sky, and thoughts have wings and can fly through the sky. Watch as each flies out of sight.

❑ 15. The sky, and thoughts are clouds. Notice each thought-cloud as it drifts by, letting it drift out of your mind.

❑ 16. A white room with two doors. Through one door, thoughts come in; through the other, thoughts go out. Watch each thought with attention and curiosity until it leaves. Let go of judgments. Let go of analyzing thoughts and of figuring out if they fit the facts. As a thought comes into your mind, say, "A thought has entered my mind."

Other: _____

Other: _____

Other: _____

Other: _____

Other: _____

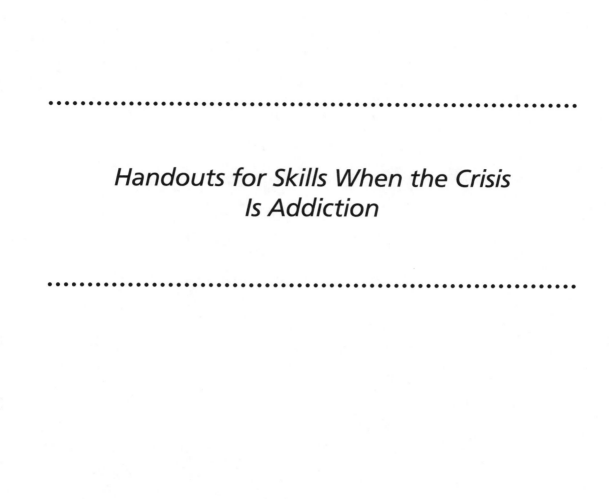

Handouts for Skills When the Crisis Is Addiction

Overview:
When the Crisis Is Addiction

Skills for backing down from addiction.
You can remember them as D, C, B, A.

D
DIALECTICAL ABSTINENCE

C
CLEAR MIND
COMMUNITY REINFORCEMENT

B
BURNING BRIDGES AND BUILDING NEW ONES

A
ALTERNATE REBELLION
ADAPTIVE DENIAL

Common Addictions

In case you thought you had no addictions, here is a list.

You are *addicted* when you are unable to stop a behavior pattern or use of substances, despite negative consequences and despite your best efforts to stop.

- ❏ Alcohol
- ❏ Attention seeking
- ❏ Avoiding: _____
- ❏ Auto racing
- ❏ Betting
- ❏ Bulimia (purging/vomiting)
- ❏ Cheating
- ❏ Coffee
- ❏ Colas
- ❏ Collecting:
  - ❏ Art
  - ❏ Coins
  - ❏ Junk
  - ❏ Clothes
  - ❏ Shoes
  - ❏ Music
  - ❏ Other: _____
  - ❏ Other: _____
- ❏ Computers
- ❏ Criminal activities
- ❏ Dieting
- ❏ Drugs (illicit and prescribed)
- ❏ Diuretics
- ❏ E-mail
- ❏ Food/eating
  - ❏ Carbohydrates
  - ❏ Chocolate
  - ❏ Specific food: _____
- ❏ Gambling
- ❏ Games/puzzles
- ❏ Gossiping
- ❏ Imagining/fantasizing
- ❏ Internet

- ❏ Internet games
- ❏ Kleptomania/stealing/shoplifting
- ❏ Lying
- ❏ Pornography
- ❏ Reckless driving
- ❏ Risky behaviors
- ❏ Self-inflicted injury/self-mutilation
- ❏ Sex
- ❏ Shopping
- ❏ Sleeping
- ❏ Smartphone apps
- ❏ Smoking/tobacco
- ❏ Social networking
- ❏ Speed
- ❏ Spiritual practices
- ❏ Sports activities:
  - ❏ Biking
  - ❏ Body building
  - ❏ Hiking/rock climbing
  - ❏ Running
  - ❏ Weight lifting
  - ❏ Other: _____
  - ❏ Other: _____
- ❏ Television
- ❏ Texting
- ❏ Vandalism
- ❏ Videos
- ❏ Video games
- ❏ Working

- ❏ Other: _____
- ❏ Other: _____
- ❏ Other: _____

Dialectical Abstinence

ABSTINENCE *(Swearing off addictive behavior)*	**vs.**	HARM REDUCTION *(Acknowledging there will be slips; minimizing the damage, but not demanding perfection)*
Pro: People who commit to abstinence stay off longer. **Con:** It takes longer for people to get back "on the wagon" once they fall off.		**Pro:** When a slip does happen, people can get back "on the wagon" faster. **Con:** People who commit to harm reduction relapse quicker.

SYNTHESIS = **DIALECTICAL ABSTINENCE**

The goal is not to engage in addictive behavior again—
in other words, to achieve complete abstinence.

However, if there is a slip, the goal is to minimize harm
and get back to abstinence as soon as possible.

> **Pros:** It works!
>
> **Cons:** It's work. You don't get a vacation.
>
> *(You're always either abstinent or working to get back to abstinence.)*

An example of expecting the best and planning for the trouble spots:
Olympic athletes must believe and behave as though they can win
every race, even though they have lost before and will lose again.

Planning for Dialectical Abstinence

Plan for Abstinence

❑ 1. Enjoy your success, but with a clear mind; plan for temptations to relapse.

❑ 2. Spend time or touch base with people who will reinforce you for abstinence.

❑ 3. Plan reinforcing activities to do instead of addictive behaviors.

❑ 4. Burn bridges: Avoid cues and high-risk situations for addictive behaviors.

❑ 5. Build new bridges: Develop images, smells, and mental activities (such as, urge surfing) to compete with information associated with craving.

❑ 6. Find alternative ways to rebel.

❑ 7. Publicly announce abstinence; deny any idea of lapsing to addiction.

Plan for Harm Reduction

❑ 1. Call your therapist, sponsor, or mentor for skills coaching.

❑ 2. Get in contact with other effective people who can help.

❑ 3. Get rid of temptations; surround yourself with cues for effective behaviors.

❑ 4. Review skills and handouts from DBT.

❑ 5. Opposite action (Emotion Regulation Handout 10) can be rehearsed to fight guilt and shame. If no other option works, go to an anonymous meeting of any sort and publicly report your lapse.

❑ 6. Building mastery and coping ahead for emotional situations (Emotion Regulation Handout 19), and checking the facts (Emotion Regulation Handout 8), can be used to fight feelings of being out of control.

❑ 7. Interpersonal skills (Interpersonal Effectiveness Handouts 5–7), such as asking for help from family, friends, sponsors, ministers, or counselors, can also be helpful. If you are isolated, help can often be found via online support groups.

❑ 8. Conduct a chain analysis to analyze what prompted the lapse (General Handouts 7, 7a).

❑ 9. Problem-solve right away to find a way to "get back on the wagon" and repair any damage you have done (Emotion Regulation Handout 12).

❑ 10. Distract yourself, self-soothe, and improve the moment.

❑ 11. Cheerlead yourself.

❑ 12. Do pros and cons of stopping addictive behaviors (Distress Tolerance Handout 5).

❑ 13. Stay away from extreme thinking. Don't let one slip turn into a disaster.

❑ 14. Recommit to 100% total abstinence.

Clear Mind

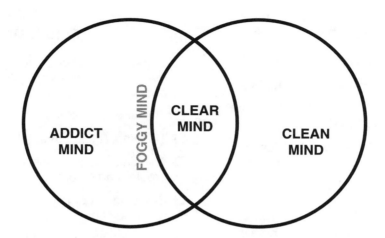

Addict mind is:

Impulsive

One-minded

Willing to do anything for a "fix"

When in ***addict mind,*** you are ruled by the addiction. The urges for habitual problem behaviors determine your thoughts, emotions, and behaviors.

Clean mind is:

Naive

Risk-taking

Oblivious to dangers

When in ***clean mind,*** you are clean but oblivious to dangers that might cue habitual problem behaviors. You believe you are invincible and immune to future temptation.

Both extremes are *DANGEROUS*!

CLEAR MIND: The safest place to be.

You are clean, but you remember addict mind.

You radically accept that relapse is ***not impossible.***

You enjoy your ***success,*** while still ***expecting urges and cues*** and ***planning*** for when you're tempted.

Behavior Patterns Characteristic of Addict Mind and of Clean Mind

ADDICT MIND

☐ Engaging in addictive behavior.

☐ Thinking, "I don't really have a problem with addiction."

☐ Thinking, "I can do a little."

☐ Thinking, "I can indulge my habit, if only on weekends."

☐ Thinking, "I can't stand this!"

☐ Glamorizing addiction.

☐ Surfing the Internet for ways to engage in addictive behaviors.

☐ Buying paraphernalia (food, drugs, videos, etc.) for addictive behavior.

☐ Selling or exchanging items related to addictive behaviors.

☐ Stealing to pay for addiction.

☐ Prostituting for money or for paraphernalia.

☐ Lying.

☐ Hiding.

☐ Isolating.

☐ Acting always busy; "Got to go!"

☐ Breaking promises.

☐ Committing crimes.

☐ Acting like a corpse.

☐ Having "no life."

☐ Acting desperate/obsessed.

☐ Not looking people in the eyes.

☐ Having poor hygiene.

☐ Avoiding doctors.

☐ Other: _____

☐ Other: _____

☐ Other: _____

CLEAN MIND

☐ Engaging in **apparently irrelevant behaviors** that in the past inevitably led to addictive behavior.

☐ Thinking, "I've learned my lesson."

☐ Thinking, "I can control the habit."

☐ Thinking, "I don't really have an addiction problem any more."

☐ Stopping or cutting back medication that helps with addiction.

☐ Being in environments where others engage in addictive behaviors.

☐ Seeing friends who are still addicted.

☐ Living with people who are addicted.

☐ Keeping addiction paraphernalia.

☐ Carrying around extra money.

☐ Being irresponsible with bills.

☐ Dressing like an addict.

☐ Not going to meetings.

☐ Not confronting the problems that fuel my addictive behaviors.

☐ Acting as if only willpower is needed.

☐ Isolating.

☐ Believing, "I can do this alone."

☐ Thinking, "I can take pain medicine/diet/ engage in addictive behavior if prescribed or advised; I don't need to say anything about my past addiction."

☐ Thinking, "I can't stand this!"

☐ Other: _____

☐ Other: _____

☐ Other: _____

Community Reinforcement

**Community reinforcement means replacing addiction reinforcers
with abstinence reinforcers.**

REINFORCING ABSTINENCE IS CRITICAL

Reinforcers in your environment play a powerful role in encouraging or discouraging addictive behaviors.

To stop addictive behavior, you have to figure out how to make a lifestyle *without* your addictive behaviors more rewarding than a lifestyle *with* your addictive behaviors.

You have to find a way to get behaviors incompatible with addictions to pay off and be rewarded by those around you.

Willpower is *not* sufficient. If it were, we would all be perfect!

REPLACE ADDICTION REINFORCERS WITH ABSTINENCE REINFORCERS

Begin a series of action steps that will increase your chances of accumulating positive events to replace addictive behavior.

❑ Search for people to spend time with who aren't addicted.

❑ Increase the number of enjoyable activities you engage in that do not involve your addiction.

❑ If you cannot decide what people or activities you like, sample a lot of different groups of people and a lot of different activities.

ABSTINENCE SAMPLING

❑ Commit to _____ days off your addiction, and observe the benefits that naturally occur.

❑ Temporarily avoid high-risk addiction triggers, and replace these with competing behaviors to get you through the sampling period.

❑ Observe all the extra positive events occurring when you are not engaging in addictive behaviors.

Note. Adapted from Meyers, R. J., & Squires, D. D. (2001, September). *The community reinforcement approach.* Retrieved from *www.bhrm.org/ guidelines/CRAmanual.pdf.* Adapted by permission of the authors.

Burning Bridges and Building New Ones

BURNING BRIDGES

Accept at the most radical level that you are not going to engage in addictive behavior again, and then move actively to cut off all addictive behavior options.

❑ **1.** Make an absolute commitment to abstinence from the addictive behavior, which is _____ (describe addictive behavior). Then walk into the garage of abstinence and **slam the garage door shut.** (Remember that the tiniest slit of space can let an entire elephant in.)

❑ **2.** List everything in your life that makes addiction possible.

❑ **3.** Get rid of these things:

  ❑ Throw out contact information of people who collude with you.

  ❑ Get rid of all possible cues and temptations.

❑ **4.** List and do everything you can that will make it hard or impossible to continue your addictive behavior.

  ❑ Ruthlessly and at every moment, tell the truth about your behavior.

  ❑ Tell all your friends and family that you have **quit.**

BUILDING NEW BRIDGES

Create visual images and smells that will compete with the information loaded into your visual and olfactory brain systems when cravings occur.

Cravings and urges are strongly related to vivid images and smells of what is craved. The stronger the imagery or smell, the stronger the craving.

  ❑ Build different images or smells to think about. Try to keep these images or smells in memory when you have an unwanted craving. For example, whenever you crave a cigarette, imagine being on the beach; see and smell it in your mind to reduce the craving.

  ❑ When you have unwanted cravings, look at moving images or surround yourself with smells unrelated to the addiction. Moving images and new smells will compete with your cravings.

  ❑ "Urge-surf" by imagining yourself on a surfboard riding the waves of your urges. Notice them coming and going, rising high, going low, and finally going away.

Alternate Rebellion and Adaptive Denial

ALTERNATE REBELLION

When addictive behaviors are a way to rebel against authority, conventions, and the boredom of not breaking rules or laws, try alternate rebellion. Alternate rebellion replaces destructive rebellion and keeps you on a path to your goals.

Examples:

- ❑ Shave your head.
- ❑ Wear crazy underwear.
- ❑ Wear unmatched shoes.
- ❑ Have secret thoughts.
- ❑ Express unpopular views.
- ❑ Do random acts of kindness.
- ❑ Vacation with your family at a nudist colony.
- ❑ Write a letter saying exactly what you want to.

- ❑ Dye your hair a wild color.
- ❑ Get a tattoo or body piercing.
- ❑ Wear clothes inside out.
- ❑ Don't bathe for a week.
- ❑ Print a slogan on a t-shirt.
- ❑ Paint your face.
- ❑ Dress up or dress down where doing so is unexpected.

ADAPTIVE DENIAL

When your mind can't tolerate craving for addictive behaviors, try adaptive denial.

❑ Give logic a break when you are doing this. Don't argue with yourself.

❑ When urges hit, deny that you want the problem behavior or substance. Convince yourself you want something other than the problem behavior. For example, reframe an urge to have a cigarette as an urge to have a flavored toothpick; an urge to have alcohol as an urge to have something sweet; or an urge to gamble as an urge to alternate rebellion (see above).

Other: _____

Other: _____

Be adamant with yourself in your denial, and engage in the alternative behavior.

❑ Put off addictive behavior. Put it off for 5 minutes, then put it off for another 5 minutes, and so on and on, each time saying, "I only have to stand this for 5 minutes." By telling yourself each day you will be abstinent for today (or each hour for just this hour, and so on), you are saying, "This is not forever. I can stand this right now."

Distress Tolerance
Worksheets

Worksheets for Crisis Survival Skills

Crisis Survival Skills

Due Date: _____   Name: _____ Week Starting: _____

Practice your crisis survival skills at least twice. Describe the crisis event; check off which skills you used for that event; and then describe how you used the skill and what happened.

CRISIS EVENT 1: Rate level of distress (0–100) Before: _____ After: _____

Prompting event for my distress (who, what, when, where): What triggered the state of crisis?

❑ **STOP**	At left, check the skills you used, and describe here:
❑ **Pros and cons**	
❑ **TIP**	
❑ **Distract with ACCEPTS**	
❑ **Self-soothe**	
❑ **IMPROVE the moment**	

Describe the outcome of using skills:

Circle a number to indicate how effective the skills were in helping you tolerate the distress and cope with the situation (keeping you from doing something to make the situation worse). Use the following scale:

I still couldn't stand the situation, even for one more minute.		*I was able to cope somewhat, at least for a little while. It helped somewhat.*		*I could use skills, tolerated distress, and resisted problem urges.*
1	2	3	4	5

CRISIS EVENT 2: Rate level of distress (0–100) Before: _____ After: _____

Prompting event for my distress (who, what, when, where): What triggered the state of crisis?

❑ **STOP**	At left, check the skills you used, and describe here:
❑ **Pros and cons**	
❑ **TIP**	
❑ **Distract with ACCEPTS**	
❑ **Self-soothe**	
❑ **IMPROVE the moment**	

Describe the outcome of using skills:

Circle effectiveness of skills:

I still couldn't stand the situation, even for one more minute.		*I was able to cope somewhat, at least for a little while. It helped somewhat.*		*I could use skills, tolerated distress, and resisted problem urges.*
1	2	3	4	5

Crisis Survival Skills

Name: _____

Week Starting: _____

Practice each crisis survival skill twice, and describe your experience as follows:

When did you practice this skill, and what did you do to practice?	What was the crisis (what prompted needing the skill)?	Amount of time practicing skill?	Rate before/after skill use			Conclusions or questions about this skills practice
			Your level of distress tolerance (0 = I can't stand it; 5 = I can definitely survive)	Emotion		
				Negative emotion intensity (0–100)	Positive emotion intensity (0–100)	
Stop:			/	/	/	
			/	/	/	
Pros and cons:			/	/	/	
			/	/	/	
TIP:			/	/	/	
			/	/	/	
Distract with ACCEPTS:			/	/	/	
			/	/	/	
Self-soothe:			/	/	/	
			/	/	/	
IMPROVE the moment:			/	/	/	
			/	/	/	

Adapted from an unpublished worksheet by Seth Axelrod, with his permission.

Crisis Survival Skills

Due Date: _____ Name: _____ Week Starting: _____

For each survival skill, write down what you did during the week, and then give a number to indicate how effective the skill was in helping you tolerate the distress and cope with the situation (keeping you from doing something to make the situation worse). Use the following scale:

I still couldn't stand the situation, even for one more minute.		*I was able to cope somewhat, at least for a little while. It helped somewhat.*		*I could use skills, tolerated distress, and resisted problem urges.*
1	**2**	**3**	**4**	**5**

Day: **STOP**

_____ /_____ Effectiveness: _____

_____ /_____ Effectiveness: _____

_____ /_____ Effectiveness: _____

Day: **Pros and cons**

_____ /_____ Effectiveness: _____

_____ /_____ Effectiveness: _____

_____ /_____ Effectiveness: _____

Day: **TIP**

_____ /_____ Effectiveness: _____

_____ /_____ Effectiveness: _____

_____ /_____ Effectiveness: _____

Day: **Distract with ACCEPTS**

_____ /_____ Effectiveness: _____

_____ /_____ Effectiveness: _____

_____ /_____ Effectiveness: _____

Day: **Self-soothe**

_____ /_____ Effectiveness: _____

_____ /_____ Effectiveness: _____

_____ /_____ Effectiveness: _____

Day: **IMPROVE the moment**

_____ /_____ Effectiveness: _____

_____ /_____ Effectiveness: _____

_____ /_____ Effectiveness: _____

Adapted from an unpublished worksheet by Seth Axelrod, with his permission.

Practicing the STOP Skill

Due Date: _____ Name: _____ Week Starting: _____

Describe two crisis situations that happened to you. Then describe your use of the STOP skill.

CRISIS EVENT 1: Rate level of distress (0–100) Before: _____ After: _____

Prompting event for my distress (who, what, when, where): What triggered the state of crisis?

Behavior you are trying to stop: _____

❑ **Stop**	At left, check the steps you used, and describe what you did here:
❑ **Take a step back**	
❑ **Observe**	
❑ **Proceed mindfully**	

Describe the outcome of using skills:

Circle a number to indicate how effective the skill was in helping you tolerate the distress and cope with the situation (keeping you from doing something to make the situation worse). Use the following scale:

I still couldn't stand the situation, even for one more minute.		I was able to cope somewhat, at least for a little while. It helped somewhat.		I could use skills, tolerated distress, and resisted problem urges.
1	2	3	4	5

CRISIS EVENT 2: Rate level of distress (0–100) Before: _____ After: _____

Prompting event for my distress (who, what, when, where): What triggered the state of crisis?

Behavior you are trying to stop: _____

❑ **Stop**	At left, check the steps you used, and describe what you did here:
❑ **Take a step back**	
❑ **Observe**	
❑ **Proceed mindfully**	

Describe the outcome of using the skills:

Circle effectiveness of the skill:

I still couldn't stand the situation, even for one more minute.		I was able to cope somewhat, at least for a little while. It helped somewhat.		I could use skills, tolerated distress, and resisted problem urges.
1	2	3	4	5

Practicing the STOP Skill

Due Date: _____   Name: _____   Week Starting: _____

Describe situations that happened to you where you used the STOP skill. Then describe how you used the STOP skill. Try to find a situation each day where you can practice your STOP skill.

Day	Crisis situation	How did you practice this skill?	Behavior stopped?	Rate before/after skill use			Conclusions or questions about this skills practice
				Your level of distress tolerance (0 = I can't stand it; 5 = I can definitely survive)	Negative emotion intensity (0–100)	Positive emotion intensity (0–100)	
					Emotion		
				—	— /	— /	
				—	— /	— /	
				—	— /	— /	
				—	— /	— /	
				—	— /	— /	
				—	— /	— /	
				—	— /	— /	

Adapted from an unpublished worksheet by Seth Axelrod, with his permission.

Pros and Cons of Acting on Crisis Urges

Due Date: _____ Name: _____ Week Starting: _____

1. Describe the *problem behavior* you are trying to stop: _____

2. List pros and cons for acting on crisis urges (including urges to act and urges to quit), and create a separate list for resisting crisis behavior by tolerating distress and using skills. Use the back of this sheet if you need more room.

3. Read the pros and cons when an urge toward the problem behavior occurs.

Problem behavior	PROS	CONS
Acting on crisis urges	1.	1.
	2.	2.
	3.	3.
	4.	4.
	5.	5.
Resisting crisis urges	1.	1.
	2.	2.
	3.	3.
	4.	4.
	5.	5.

Identify which pros and cons are short-term (just for today) or long-term (beyond today). Then ask your Wise Mind: Would you rather have a good day or a good life? Make a mindful choice about your behavior.

If this worksheet helps you choose skillful behavior over crisis behavior, be sure to keep it where you can find it and review it again when you are in crisis.

Adapted from an unpublished worksheet by Seth Axelrod, with his permission.

Pros and Cons of Acting on Crisis Urges

Due Date: _____ Name: _____ Week Starting: _____

1. Describe the *problem behavior* you are trying to stop: _____

2. List pros and cons for acting on crisis urges (including urges to act and urges to quit), and create a separate list for resisting crisis behavior by tolerating distress and using skills. Use the back of this sheet if you need more room.

3. Read the pros and cons when an urge toward the problem behavior occurs.

Problem behavior	Acting on crisis urges	Resisting crisis urges
PROS	1.	1.
	2.	2.
	3.	3.
	4.	4.
	5.	5.
CONS	1.	1.
	2.	2.
	3.	3.
	4.	4.
	5.	5.

Identify which pros and cons are short-term (just for today) or long-term (beyond today). Then ask your Wise Mind: Would you rather have a good day or a good life? Make a mindful choice about your behavior.

If this worksheet helps you choose skillful behavior over crisis behavior, be sure to keep it where you can find it and review it again when you are in crisis.

Adapted from an unpublished worksheet by Seth Axelrod, with his permission.

375

Changing Body Chemistry with TIP Skills

Due Date: _____ Name: _____ Week Starting: _____

Describe the situation you were in when you chose to practice each skill. Rate both your emotional arousal and distress tolerance before and after using the TIP skill. Describe what you actually did. Use the back of this sheet if necessary.

T

CHANGING MY FACIAL TEMPERATURE

Used cold water to change emotions

Situation: _____

Arousal (0–100) Before: _____ After: _____

Distress tolerance (0 = I can't stand it; 100 = I can definitely survive) Before: _____ After: _____

What I did (describe): _____

_____

I

INTENSE EXERCISE

Situation: _____

Arousal (0–100) Before: _____ After: _____

Distress tolerance (0 = I can't stand it; 100 = I can definitely survive) Before: _____ After: _____

What I did (describe): _____

_____

P

PACED BREATHING

Situation: _____

Arousal (0–100) Before: _____ After: _____

Distress tolerance (0 = I can't stand it; 100 = I can definitely survive) Before: _____ After: _____

What I did (describe): _____

_____

PAIRED MUSCLE RELAXATION

Situation: _____

Arousal (0–100) Before: _____ After: _____

Distress tolerance (0 = I can't stand it; 100 = I can definitely survive) Before: _____ After: _____

What I did (describe): _____

_____

Paired Muscle Relaxation

Due Date: _____ Name: _____ Week Starting: _____

Practice **Paired Muscle Relaxation** (tensing your body muscles and then letting go of tension completely as you breathe out). Practice as many times a day as you can at first until you notice that when you exhale, our body automatically relaxes on its own. At this point, you have paired breathing out with relaxation. Once that happens, continue practicing but not as often.

Practice paired muscle relaxation as many times a day as you can, and describe your experience below. Check the type of practice you did: individual muscles, muscle groups, or all of your muscles at once.

Day	Number of times *practiced* paired muscle relaxation	Average level of relaxation before/after (0–100)	Number of times *used skill* when tense or overwhelmed	Average level of relaxation before/after (0–100)	Check which muscles you tensed and relaxed (check more than one if necessary)
		/		/	❑ Individual muscles ❑ Groups ❑ All at once
		/		/	❑ Individual muscles ❑ Groups ❑ All at once
		/		/	❑ Individual muscles ❑ Groups ❑ All at once
		/		/	❑ Individual muscles ❑ Groups ❑ All at once
		/		/	❑ Individual muscles ❑ Groups ❑ All at once
		/		/	❑ Individual muscles ❑ Groups ❑ All at once

Describe your experience:

Conclusions about practice and/or questions about this skills practice:

(Distress Tolerance Handout 6c)

Effective Rethinking and Paired Relaxation

Due Date: _____   Name: _____ Week Starting: _____

Step 1. Describe one typical **prompting event** for distress in your life: What led up to what? What is it about this event that is a problem for you? Be very specific in your answers. Use describing skills. Check the facts.

Step 2. Ask: "What must I be telling myself (or what are my **interpretations and thoughts**) about this event that contributes to my stress?" **Write them down.**

Step 3. Rethink the thoughts that lead to distress. Rethinking involves reevaluating the situation and its meaning in ways that counteract stress-producing thoughts and thereby reduce stress responses. **Write down** as many effective thoughts as you can to replace the stressful thoughts.

Step 4. Did you practice **in your imagination** effective rethinking of a stressful situation this week? Yes _____ No _____

   If you engaged in rethinking, did it reduce fear of the situation happening again? (0–5, 0 = not at all; 5 = very much): _____

What effective thoughts did you use to replace stress-causing thoughts?

Rate average level of relaxation (0–100): Before _____ After _____

Step 5. Did you practice **rethinking plus paired relaxation**? Yes _____ No _____

   If you engaged in rethinking plus paired relaxation, did it help you reduce your stress? (0–5, 0 = not at all; 5 = very much): _____

What effective thoughts did you use to replace stress-causing thoughts?

Comments:

Distracting with Wise Mind ACCEPTS

Due Date: _____ Name: _____ Week Starting: _____

Describe two crisis situations that happened to you. Then describe your use of the ACCEPTS skills.

CRISIS EVENT 1: Rate level of distress (0–100) Before: _____ After: _____

> **Prompting event** for my distress (who, what, when, where): What triggered the state of crisis?

❑ **A**ctivities
❑ **C**ontributions
❑ **C**omparisons
❑ **E**motions
❑ **P**ushing away
❑ **T**houghts
❑ **S**ensations

> At left, check the skills you used, and describe here:

> Describe the outcome of using skills:

Circle a number to indicate how effective the skills were in helping you tolerate the distress and cope with the situation (keeping you from doing something to make the situation worse). Use the following scale:

I still couldn't stand the situation, even for one more minute.		*I was able to cope somewhat, at least for a little while. It helped somewhat.*		*I could use skills, tolerated distress, and resisted problem urges.*
1	**2**	**3**	**4**	**5**

CRISIS EVENT 2: Rate level of distress (0–100) Before: _____ After: _____

> **Prompting event** for my distress (who, what, when, where): What triggered the state of crisis?

❑ **A**ctivities
❑ **C**ontributions
❑ **C**omparisons
❑ **E**motions
❑ **P**ushing away
❑ **T**houghts
❑ **S**ensations

> At left, check the skills you used, and describe here:

> Describe the outcome of using skills:

Circle effectiveness of skills:

I still couldn't stand the situation, even for one more minute.		*I was able to cope somewhat, at least for a little while. It helped somewhat.*		*I could use skills, tolerated distress, and resisted problem urges.*
1	**2**	**3**	**4**	**5**

Distracting with Wise Mind ACCEPTS

Due Date: _____   Name: _____   Week Starting: _____

Practice each distraction skill twice, and describe your experience as follows:

When did you practice this skill, and what did you do to practice?	What was the crisis (what prompted needing the skill)?	How much time passed in doing this skill?	Rate before/after skill use			Conclusions or questions about this skills practice
			Distress tolerance (0 = I can't stand it; 5 = I can definitely survive)	Negative emotion intensity (0–100)	Positive emotion intensity (0–100)	
					Emotion	
Activities:			/	/	/	
			/	/	/	
Contributions:			/	/	/	
			/	/	/	
Comparisons:			/	/	/	
			/	/	/	
Emotions:			/	/	/	
			/	/	/	
Pushing away:			/	/	/	
			/	/	/	
Thoughts:			/	/	/	
			/	/	/	
Sensations:			/	/	/	
			/	/	/	

Adapted from an unpublished worksheet by Seth Axelrod, with his permission.

Distracting with Wise Mind ACCEPTS

Due Date: _____   Name: _____   Week Starting: _____

For each ACCEPTS skill, write down what you did during the week, and write down a number to indicate how effective the skill was in helping you tolerate the distress and cope with the situation (keeping you from doing something to make the situation worse). Use the following scale:

I still couldn't stand the situation, even for one more minute.		I was able to cope somewhat, at least for a little while. It helped somewhat.		I could use skills, tolerated distress, and resisted problem urges.
1	2	3	4	5

Day: **ACTIVITIES**
_____ /_____ Effectiveness: _____
_____ /_____ Effectiveness: _____
_____ /_____ Effectiveness: _____

Day: **CONTRIBUTIONS**
_____ /_____ Effectiveness: _____
_____ /_____ Effectiveness: _____
_____ /_____ Effectiveness: _____

Day: **COMPARISONS**
_____ /_____ Effectiveness: _____
_____ /_____ Effectiveness: _____
_____ /_____ Effectiveness: _____

Day: **EMOTIONS**
_____ /_____ Effectiveness: _____
_____ /_____ Effectiveness: _____
_____ /_____ Effectiveness: _____

Day: **PUSHING AWAY**
_____ /_____ Effectiveness: _____
_____ /_____ Effectiveness: _____
_____ /_____ Effectiveness: _____

Day: **THOUGHTS**
_____ /_____ Effectiveness: _____
_____ /_____ Effectiveness: _____
_____ /_____ Effectiveness: _____

Day: **SENSATIONS**
_____ /_____ Effectiveness: _____
_____ /_____ Effectiveness: _____
_____ /_____ Effectiveness: _____

381

Self-Soothing

Due Date: _____ Name: _____ Week Starting: _____

Describe two crisis situations that happened to you. Then describe your use of the self-soothing skills.

CRISIS EVENT 1: Rate level of distress (0–100) Before: _____ After: _____

Prompting event for my distress (who, what, when, where): What triggered the state of crisis?

❑ **Vision**
❑ **Hearing**
❑ **Smell**
❑ **Taste**
❑ **Touch**

At left, check the skills you used, and describe here:

Describe the outcome of using skills:

Circle a number to indicate how effective the skills were in helping you tolerate the distress and cope with the situation (keeping you from doing something to make the situation worse). Use the following scale:

I still couldn't stand the situation, even for one more minute.		*I was able to cope somewhat, at least for a little while. It helped somewhat.*		*I could use skills, tolerated distress, and resisted problem urges.*
1	**2**	**3**	**4**	**5**

CRISIS EVENT 2: Rate level of distress (0–100) Before: _____ After: _____

Prompting event for my distress (who, what, when, where): What triggered the state of crisis?

❑ **Vision**
❑ **Hearing**
❑ **Smell**
❑ **Taste**
❑ **Touch**

At left, check the skills you used, and describe here:

Describe the outcome of using skills:

Circle effectiveness of skills:

I still couldn't stand the situation, even for one more minute.		*I was able to cope somewhat, at least for a little while. It helped somewhat.*		*I could use skills, tolerated distress, and resisted problem urges.*
1	**2**	**3**	**4**	**5**

Self-Soothing

Due Date: _____   Name: _____   Week Starting: _____

Practice each self-soothing skill twice, and describe your experience as follows:

When did you practice this skill, and what did you do to practice?	What was going on that was painful or stressful (if anything)?	How much time passed in doing this skill?	Rate before/after skill use			Conclusions or questions about this skills practice
			Distress tolerance (0 = I can't stand it; 5 = I can definitely survive)	Emotion		
				Negative emotion intensity (0–100)	Positive emotion intensity (0–100)	
Vision:			___ / ___	___ / ___	___ / ___	
			___ / ___	___ / ___	___ / ___	
Hearing:			___ / ___	___ / ___	___ / ___	
			___ / ___	___ / ___	___ / ___	
Smell:			___ / ___	___ / ___	___ / ___	
			___ / ___	___ / ___	___ / ___	
Taste:			___ / ___	___ / ___	___ / ___	
			___ / ___	___ / ___	___ / ___	
Touch:			___ / ___	___ / ___	___ / ___	

Adapted from an unpublished worksheet by Seth Axelrod, with his permission.

Self-Soothing

Due Date: _____   Name: _____ Week Starting: _____

For each self-soothing skill, write down what you did during the week, and write down a number to indicate how effective the skill was in helping you tolerate the distress and cope with the situation (keeping you from doing something to make the situation worse). Use the following scale:

I still couldn't stand the situation, even for one more minute.		I was able to cope somewhat, at least for a little while. It helped somewhat.		I could use skills, tolerated distress, and resisted problem urges.
1	**2**	**3**	**4**	**5**

Day: **VISION**

_____ /_____ Effectiveness: ____

_____ /_____ Effectiveness: ____

_____ /_____ Effectiveness: ____

_____ /_____ Effectiveness: ____

Day: **HEARING**

_____ /_____ Effectiveness: ____

_____ /_____ Effectiveness: ____

_____ /_____ Effectiveness: ____

_____ /_____ Effectiveness: ____

Day: **SMELL**

_____ /_____ Effectiveness: ____

_____ /_____ Effectiveness: ____

_____ /_____ Effectiveness: ____

_____ /_____ Effectiveness: ____

Day: **TASTE**

_____ /_____ Effectiveness: ____

_____ /_____ Effectiveness: ____

_____ /_____ Effectiveness: ____

_____ /_____ Effectiveness: ____

Day: **TOUCH**

_____ /_____ Effectiveness: ____

_____ /_____ Effectiveness: ____

_____ /_____ Effectiveness: ____

_____ /_____ Effectiveness: ____

Body Scan Meditation, Step by Step

Due Date: _____ Name: _____ Week Starting: _____

Practice as many times as you can. Check whether you practiced alone, listening to a recording, watching YouTube, or being guided by a person.

Day	Describe your experience		How much time passed doing this skiill?	Rate before and after body scan		
					Emotion	
				Distress tolerance (0 = I can't stand it; 5 = I can definitely survive)	Negative emotion intensity (0–100)	Positive emotion intensity (0–100)
1	☐ Alone	☐ Recording		/	/	/
	☐ Person guiding	☐ YouTube				
2	☐ Alone	☐ Recording		/	/	/
	☐ Person guiding	☐ YouTube				
3	☐ Alone	☐ Recording		/	/	/
	☐ Person guiding	☐ YouTube				
4	☐ Alone	☐ Recording		/	/	/
	☐ Person guiding	☐ YouTube				
5	☐ Alone	☐ Recording		/	/	/
	☐ Person guiding	☐ YouTube				

Conclusions or questions about this skills practice:

Adapted from an unpublished worksheet by Seth Axelrod, with his permission.

IMPROVE the Moment

Due Date: _____ Name: _____ Week Starting: _____

Describe two crisis situations that happened to you. Then describe your use of the IMPROVE skills.

CRISIS EVENT 1: Rate level of distress (0–100) Before: _____ After: _____

Prompting event for my distress (who, what, when, where): What triggered the state of crisis?

❑ **I**magery
❑ **M**eaning
❑ **P**rayer
❑ **R**elaxation
❑ **O**ne thing
❑ **V**acation
❑ **E**ncouragement

At left, check the skills you used, and describe here:

Describe the outcome of using skills:

Circle a number to indicate how effective the skills were in helping you tolerate the distress and cope with the situation (keeping you from doing something to make the situation worse). Use the following scale:

I still couldn't stand the situation, even for one more minute.		*I was able to cope somewhat, at least for a little while. It helped somewhat.*		*I could use skills, tolerated distress, and resisted problem urges.*
1	**2**	**3**	**4**	**5**

CRISIS EVENT 2: Rate level of distress (0–100) Before: _____ After: _____

Prompting event for my distress (who, what, when, where): What triggered the state of crisis?

❑ **I**magery
❑ **M**eaning
❑ **P**rayer
❑ **R**elaxation
❑ **O**ne thing
❑ **V**acation
❑ **E**ncouragement

At left, check the skills you used, and describe here:

Describe the outcome of using skills:

Circle effectiveness of skills:

I still couldn't stand the situation, even for one more minute.		*I was able to cope somewhat, at least for a little while. It helped somewhat.*		*I could use skills, tolerated distress, and resisted problem urges.*
1	**2**	**3**	**4**	**5**

IMPROVE the Moment

Due Date: _____ Name: _____ Week Starting: _____

Practice each IMPROVE skill twice, and describe your experience as follows:

When did you practice this skill, and what did you do to practice?	What was going on that was painful or stressful (if anything)?	How much time passed in doing this skill?	Rate before/after skill use			Conclusions or questions about this skills practice
			Distress tolerance (0 = I can't stand it; 5 = I can definitely survive)	Emotion		
				Negative emotion intensity (0–100)	Positive emotion intensity (0–100)	
Imagery:			__/__	__/__	__/__	
			__/__	__/__	__/__	
Meaning:			__/__	__/__	__/__	
			__/__	__/__	__/__	
Prayer:			__/__	__/__	__/__	
			__/__	__/__	__/__	
Relaxation:			__/__	__/__	__/__	
			__/__	__/__	__/__	
One thing:			__/__	__/__	__/__	
			__/__	__/__	__/__	
Vacation:			__/__	__/__	__/__	
			__/__	__/__	__/__	
Encouragement:			__/__	__/__	__/__	
			__/__	__/__	__/__	

Adapted from an unpublished worksheet by Seth Axelrod, with his permission.

IMPROVE the Moment

Due Date: _____ Name: _____ Week Starting: _____

For each IMPROVE skill, write down what you did during the week, and write down a number to indicate how effective the skill was in helping you tolerate the distress and cope with the situation (keeping you from doing something to make the situation worse). Use the following scale:

I still couldn't stand the situation, even for one more minute.		*I was able to cope somewhat, at least for a little while. It helped somewhat.*		*I could use skills, tolerated distress, and resisted problem urges.*
1	**2**	**3**	**4**	**5**

Day: <u>I</u>MAGERY

_____ /_____ Effectiveness: _____

_____ /_____ Effectiveness: _____

_____ /_____ Effectiveness: _____

Day: <u>M</u>EANING

_____ /_____ Effectiveness: _____

_____ /_____ Effectiveness: _____

_____ /_____ Effectiveness: _____

Day: <u>P</u>RAYER

_____ /_____ Effectiveness: _____

_____ /_____ Effectiveness: _____

_____ /_____ Effectiveness: _____

Day: <u>R</u>ELAXATION

_____ /_____ Effectiveness: _____

_____ /_____ Effectiveness: _____

_____ /_____ Effectiveness: _____

Day: <u>O</u>NE THING IN THE MOMENT

_____ /_____ Effectiveness: _____

_____ /_____ Effectiveness: _____

_____ /_____ Effectiveness: _____

Day: <u>V</u>ACATION

_____ /_____ Effectiveness: _____

_____ /_____ Effectiveness: _____

_____ /_____ Effectiveness: _____

Day: <u>E</u>NCOURAGEMENT

_____ /_____ Effectiveness: _____

_____ /_____ Effectiveness: _____

_____ /_____ Effectiveness: _____

Worksheets for Reality Acceptance Skills

Reality Acceptance Skills

Due Date: _____ Name: _____ Week Starting: _____

Check off two reality acceptance skills to practice this week during a stressful situation:

- ❑ Radical acceptance
- ❑ Turning the mind
- ❑ Willingness

- ❑ Half-smiling
- ❑ Willing hands
- ❑ Mindfulness of current thoughts

Skill 1. Describe the situation and how you practiced the skill:

_____

_____

How effective was the skill in helping you cope with the situation (keeping you from doing something to make the situation worse)? Circle a number below.

I still couldn't stand the situation, even for one more minute.		I was able to cope somewhat, at least for a little while. It helped somewhat.		I could use skills, tolerated distress, and resisted problem urges.
1	2	3	4	5

Did this skill help you cope with uncomfortable emotions or urges, *or* avoid conflict of any kind? Circle YES or NO.

Describe how the skill helped or did not help: _____

_____

Skill 2. Describe the situation and how you practiced the skill:

_____

_____

How effective was the skill in helping you cope with the situation (keeping you from doing something to make the situation worse)? Circle a number below.

I still couldn't stand the situation, even for one more minute.		I was able to cope somewhat, at least for a little while. It helped somewhat.		I could use skills, tolerated distress, and resisted problem urges.
1	2	3	4	5

Did this skill help you cope with uncomfortable emotions or urges, *or* avoid conflict of any kind? Circle YES or NO.

Describe how the skill helped or did not help: _____

_____

Reality Acceptance Skills

Due Date: _____ Name: _____ Week Starting: _____

Practice each reality acceptance skill twice, and describe your experience as follows:

When did you practice this skill, and what did you do to practice?	What was going on that you had trouble accepting (if anything)?	How long did you practice accepting?	Rate before/after skill use			Conclusions or questions about this skills practice
			Acceptance (0 = none at all; 5 = I am at peace with this)	Emotion		
				Negative emotion intensity (0–100)	Positive emotion intensity (0–100)	
Radical acceptance:			/	/	/	
			/	/	/	
Turning the mind:			/	/	/	
			/	/	/	
Willingness:			/	/	/	
			/	/	/	
Half-smiling:			/	/	/	
			/	/	/	
Willing hands:			/	/	/	
			/	/	/	
Mindfulness of current thoughts:			/	/	/	
			/	/	/	

Adapted from an unpublished worksheet by Seth Axelrod, with his permission.

Reality Acceptance Skills

Due Date: _____ Name: _____ Week Starting: _____

For each reality acceptance skill, describe the skill you used during the week, and circle a number (0–5) indicating your own experience of acceptance of yourself, your life, or events outside yourself. Use the following scale:

No acceptance; I am in complete denial and/or rebellion		I was able to accept somewhat or for a little while.		Complete acceptance; I am at peace with this.
1	2	3	4	5

Day: **RADICAL ACCEPTANCE** (describe what and how often you practiced)

_____ /_____ Effectiveness: ____

_____ /_____ Effectiveness: ____

_____ /_____ Effectiveness: ____

Day: **TURNING THE MIND** (describe the cross-road you were at, and what you chose)

_____ /_____ Effectiveness: ____

_____ /_____ Effectiveness: ____

_____ /_____ Effectiveness: ____

Day: **WILLINGNESS** (describe the situation, what you were willful about, and how you practiced)

_____ /_____ Effectiveness: ____

_____ /_____ Effectiveness: ____

_____ /_____ Effectiveness: ____

Day: **HALF-SMILING** (describe the situation and how you practiced)

_____ /_____ Effectiveness: ____

_____ /_____ Effectiveness: ____

_____ /_____ Effectiveness: ____

Day: **WILLING HANDS** (describe the situation and how you practiced)

_____ /_____ Effectiveness: ____

_____ /_____ Effectiveness: ____

_____ /_____ Effectiveness: ____

Day: **MINDFULNESS OF CURRENT THOUGHTS** (describe what thoughts were going through your mind and *how* you observed your thoughts)

_____ /_____ Effectiveness: ____

_____ /_____ Effectiveness: ____

_____ /_____ Effectiveness: ____

Radical Acceptance

Due Date: _____   Name: _____ Week Starting: _____

FIGURE OUT WHAT YOU NEED TO RADICALLY ACCEPT

1. Make a list of two **very important** things in your life right now that you need to radically accept. Then give each one a number indicating how much you accept this part of yourself or your life: from 0 (no acceptance, I am in complete denial and/or rebellion) to 5 (complete acceptance, I am at peace with this). *Note:* if you have already completed this section, you don't need to do it again unless things have changed.

   What I need to accept   (Acceptance, 0–5)

   1. _____ (_____)

   2. _____ (_____)

2. Make a list of two **less important** things in your life you are having trouble accepting this week. Then rate your acceptance just as you did above.

   What I need to accept   (Acceptance, 0–5)

   1. _____ (_____)

   2. _____ (_____)

REFINE YOUR LIST

3. Review your two lists above. **Check the facts.** Check for interpretations and opinions. Make sure that what you are trying to accept is in fact the case. **Check for judgments.** Avoid "good," "bad," and judgmental language. Rewrite any items above if needed so that they are **factual and nonjudgmental.**

PRACTICE RADICAL ACCEPTANCE

4. Choose one item from the very important list and one item from the less important list to practice on.

   1. _____

   2. _____

5. Focus your mind on each of these facts or events separately, allowing your Wise Mind to radically accept that these *are* facts of your life. *Check off* any of the following exercises that you did.

   ❑ Observed that I was questioning or fighting reality.
   ❑ Reminded myself that reality is what it is.
   ❑ Considered the causes of the reality, and nonjudgmentally accepted that causes exist.
   ❑ Practiced accepting all the way with my whole being (mind, body, spirit).
   ❑ Practiced opposite action.
   ❑ Coped ahead with events that seemed unacceptable.

   ❑ Attended to my body sensations as I thought about what I need to accept.
   ❑ Allowed myself to experience disappointment, sadness, or grief.
   ❑ Acknowledged that life can be worth living even when there is pain.
   ❑ Did pros and cons of accepting versus denial and rejection.
   ❑ Other: _____
   _____

6. Rate your degree of acceptance after practicing radical acceptance (0–5): _____

Practicing Radical Acceptance

Due Date: _____ Name: _____ Week Starting: _____

Practice each skill twice, and describe and rate your experience below.

When did you practice this skill, and what did you do to practice?	How long did you practice accepting?	Rate before/after skill use			Conclusions or questions about this skills practice
		Acceptance (0 = none at all; 5 = I am at peace with this)	Emotion		
			Negative emotion intensity (0–100)	Positive emotion intensity (0–100)	
What was going on that you had trouble accepting (if anything)?					
Considered causes of the reality:		/	/	/	
		/	/	/	
Practiced with my whole self:		/	/	/	
		/	/	/	
Practiced opposite action:		/	/	/	
		/	/	/	
Practiced coping ahead:		/	/	/	
		/	/	/	
Attended to body sensations:		/	/	/	
		/	/	/	
Allowed disappointment/grieving:		/	/	/	
		/	/	/	
Acknowledged life as worth living:		/	/	/	
		/	/	/	
Did pros and cons:		/	/	/	
		/	/	/	

Adapted from an unpublished worksheet by Seth Axelrod, with his permission.

Turning the Mind, Willingness, Willfulness

Due Date: _____ Name: _____ Week Starting: _____

Practice each skill, and rate your level of acceptance of reality as it is before and after: from 0 (no acceptance at all) to 5 (I'm at peace with this). List what you tried specifically under the rating.

Turning the Mind: Acceptance   Before: _____ After: _____

OBSERVE not accepting. What did you observe? What were you having trouble accepting?

MAKE AN INNER COMMITMENT to accept what feels unacceptable. How did you do this?

Describe your **PLAN FOR CATCHING YOURSELF** the next time you drift from acceptance.

WILLINGNESS (rate 0–5): Acceptance   Before: _____ After: _____
Willfulness   Before: _____ After: _____

Describe **EFFECTIVE BEHAVIOR** you did to move forward toward a goal.

NOTICE WILLFULNESS. Describe how you are not participating effectively in the world as it is, or how you are not doing something you know needs to be done to move toward a goal.

Describe how you **PRACTICED RADICALLY ACCEPTING YOUR WILLFULNESS.**

MAKE AN INNER COMMITMENT to accept what feels unacceptable. How did you do this?

Describe what you did that was **WILLING.**

Half-Smiling and Willing Hands

Due Date: _____ Name: _____ Week Starting: _____

Describe your practice with half-smiling and willing hands this past week. Practice each day at least once. Practice both when you are not emotionally distressed and when you are distressed.

Check off any of the following exercises that you did.

- ❑ 1. Half-smiled when I first woke up in the morning.
- ❑ 2. Half-smiled during my free moments.
- ❑ 3. Half-smiled with willing hands while I was listening to music.
- ❑ 4. Half-smiled with willing hands when I was irritated.
- ❑ 5. Half-smiled in a lying-down position.
- ❑ 6. Half-smiled in a sitting position.
- ❑ 7. Half-smiled when I was walking down the street.

- ❑ 8. Half-smiled with willing hands when my feelings were hurt.
- ❑ 9. Half-smiled with willing hands when I did not want to accept something.
- ❑ 10. Half-smiled with willing hands when I started getting really angry.
- ❑ 11. Half-smiled when I had negative thoughts.
- ❑ 12. Half-smiled when I couldn't sleep.
- ❑ 13. Half-smiled with another person.
- ❑ 14. Other: _____
  _____

Describe practicing half-smiling and willing hands.

1. Situation: _____

Describe strategies you used or give numbers from above: _____

Circle how effective this was at helping you be more mindful and less reactive:

1	2	3	4	5
Not effective		*Somewhat effective*		*Very effective*

2. Situation: _____

Describe strategies you used or give numbers from above: _____

Circle how effective this was at helping you be more mindful and less reactive:

1	2	3	4	5
Not effective		*Somewhat effective*		*Very effective*

3. Situation: _____

Describe strategies you used or give numbers from above: _____

Circle how effective this was at helping you be more mindful and less reactive:

1	2	3	4	5
Not effective		*Somewhat effective*		*Very effective*

Practicing Half-Smiling and Willing Hands

Due Date: _____ Name: _____ Week Starting: _____

Practice half-smiling/willing hands twice each day. Describe what you did to practice, and what you were trying to accept. (See Distress Tolerance Worksheet 11 for ideas.)

What did you do to practice allowing your thoughts?	What were you having trouble accepting (if any)?	How much time passed in doing this skill?	Rate before/after skill use			Conclusions or questions about this skills practice
			Acceptance (0 = none at all; 5 = I am at peace with this)	Emotion		
				Negative emotion intensity (0–100)	Positive emotion intensity (0–100)	
Mon			/	/	/	
Tues			/	/	/	
Wed			/	/	/	
Thurs			/	/	/	
Fri			/	/	/	
Sat			/	/	/	
Sun			/	/	/	

Adapted from an unpublished worksheet by Seth Axelrod, with his permission.

Mindfulness of Current Thoughts

Due Date: _____ Name: _____ Week Starting: _____

Describe your efforts to observe your thoughts in the past week. Practice observing thoughts each day at least once. Don't focus just on thoughts that are painful, anxiety-provoking, or full of anger; also observe and be mindful of pleasant or neutral thoughts. For each thought, first practice saying, "The thought [describe thought] went through my mind." Then practice one or more strategies to observe and let go of thoughts.

Check off any of the following exercises that you did.

- ❑ 1. Used words and voice tone to say a thought over and over; as fast as I could; very, very slowly; in a voice different from mine; as a dialogue on a TV comedy show; or as singing.
- ❑ 2. Relaxed my face and body imagining accepting my thoughts as sensations of my brain.
- ❑ 3. Imagined what I would do if I stopped believing everything I think.
- ❑ 4. Rehearsed in my mind what I would do if I did not view my thoughts as facts.
- ❑ 5. Practiced loving my thoughts as they went through my mind.
- ❑ 6. Refocused my mind on sensations I was avoiding by worrying or catastrophizing.
- ❑ 7. Allowed my thoughts to come and go as I focused on observing my breath coming in and out.
- ❑ 8. Labeled the thought as a thought, saying, "The thought [describe thought] arose in my mind."
- ❑ 9. Asked, "Where did the thought come from?" and watched my mind to find out.
- ❑ 10. Stepped back from my mind, as if I was on top of a mountain.
- ❑ 11. Shuttled back and forth between scanning for physical sensations and scanning for thoughts.
- ❑ 12. Imagined that in my mind thoughts were coming down a conveyor belt; were boats on a river; were train cars on a railroad track; were written on leaves flowing down a river; had wings and could fly away; were clouds floating in the sky; or were going in and out of the doors of my mind. (Underline the image you used.)
- ❑ 13. Other:_____

Describe thoughts you were mindful of during the week. State just each thought as it went through your mind.

---

1. Thought: _____
Describe strategies you used or give numbers from above: _____
Circle how effective was this at helping you be more mindful and less reactive:

1	2	3	4	5
Not effective		*Somewhat effective*		*Very effective*

---

2. Thought: _____
Describe strategies you used or give numbers from above: _____
Circle how effective was this at helping you be more mindful and less reactive:

1	2	3	4	5
Not effective		*Somewhat effective*		*Very effective*

---

3. Thought: _____
Describe strategies you used or give numbers from above: _____
Circle how effective was this at helping you be more mindful and less reactive:

1	2	3	4	5
Not effective		*Somewhat effective*		*Very effective*

Practicing Mindfulness of Thoughts

Due Date: _____   Name: _____   Week Starting: _____

Practice allowing the mind twice each day. Describe what strategy you used to allow your thoughts, and what thoughts you had. (See Distress Tolerance Worksheet 12 for ideas.) Rate your experience below.

What did you do to practice allowing your thoughts?	What were you having trouble accepting (if any)?	How much time passed in doing this skill?	Rate before/after skill use			Conclusions or questions about this skills practice
			Acceptance (0 = none at all; 5 = I am at peace with this)	Emotion		
				Negative emotion intensity (0–100)	Positive emotion intensity (0–100)	
Mon			/	/	/	
Tues			/	/	/	
Wed			/	/	/	
Thurs			/	/	/	
Fri			/	/	/	
Sat			/	/	/	
Sun			/	/	/	

Adapted from an unpublished worksheet by Seth Axelrod, with his permission.

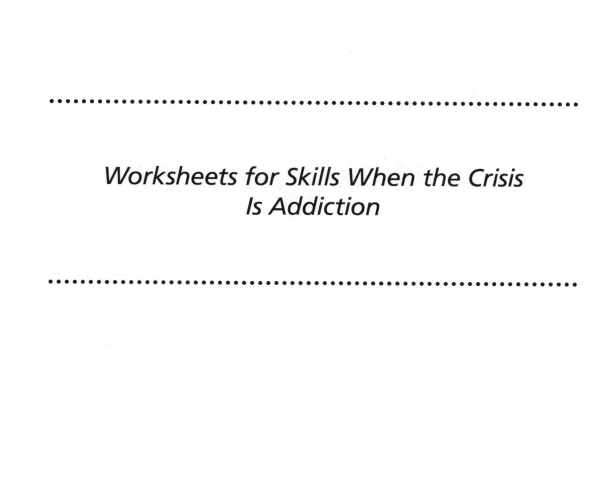

Worksheets for Skills When the Crisis Is Addiction

Skills When the Crisis Is Addiction

Due Date: _____ Name: _____ Week Starting: _____

Check off two skills for backing down from addiction to practice this week during a stressful situation:

- ❏ Plan for abstinence
- ❏ Plan for harm reduction
- ❏ Practice clear mind
- ❏ Search for abstinence reinforcers
- ❏ Increase non-addicting pleasant events

- ❏ Sample abstinence for _____ days
- ❏ Burn bridges
- ❏ Build new bridges
- ❏ Practice alternate rebellion
- ❏ Practice adaptive denial

Skill 1. Describe the situation and how you practiced the skill:

_____

_____

How effective was the skill in helping you cope with the situation (keeping you from doing something to make the situation worse)? Circle a number below.

I still couldn't stand the situation, even for one more minute.		*I was able to cope somewhat, at least for a little while. It helped somewhat.*		*I could use skills, tolerated distress, and resisted problem urges.*
1	**2**	**3**	**4**	**5**

Did this skill help you cope with uncomfortable emotions or urges, *or* avoid conflict of any kind? Circle YES or NO.

Describe how the skill helped or did not help: _____

_____

Skill 2. Describe the situation and how you practiced the skill:

_____

_____

How effective was the skill in helping you cope with the situation (keeping you from doing something to make the situation worse)? Circle a number below.

I still couldn't stand the situation, even for one more minute.		*I was able to cope somewhat, at least for a little while. It helped somewhat.*		*I could use skills, tolerated distress, and resisted problem urges.*
1	**2**	**3**	**4**	**5**

Did this skill help you cope with uncomfortable emotions or urges, *or* avoid conflict of any kind? Circle YES or NO.

Describe how the skill helped or did not help: _____

_____

Planning for Dialectical Abstinence

Due Date: _____ Name: _____ Week Starting: _____

Problem Behavior: _____

Check each activity and describe what you did.

PLAN FOR ABSTINENCE

To maximize the chances I'll stop _____, I need to aim for abstinence.

❑ Plan activities to do instead of problem behaviors (e.g., work, find a hobby, go to a support meeting, volunteer). These will include:

_____

_____

❑ Spend time or touch base with people who will reinforce my *not* engaging in problem behaviors and my engaging in effective behaviors (e.g., effective friends or family members, co-workers, employers, my therapist, people from group). These people include:

_____

_____

❑ Remind myself of reasons to stay abstinent and be effective (e.g., to reach long-term goals, to keep/get relationship, to save money, to avoid shame). These include:

_____

_____

_____

❑ Burn bridges with people who represent a temptation (e.g., lose their numbers, unfriend them, tell them to stop contacting me, make them not want to hang out with me). These people include:

_____

_____

❑ Avoid cues for problem behaviors. Cues include:

_____

_____

_____

*(**continued on next page**)*

❑ Use skills (things to do to avoid urges, interpersonal effectiveness, distress tolerance, emotion regulation, mindfulness). The most useful skills for me include:

_____

_____

_____

❑ Find alternative ways to rebel. These include:

_____

_____

_____

❑ Publicly announce I've embraced abstinence and effective behavior.

PLAN FOR HARM REDUCTION

If I have a slip, I don't want the slip to turn into a slide. To avoid a slide, I must have plans to regain my balance and get back to abstinence and effectiveness.

❑ Call my therapist, sponsor, or mentor for skills coaching. His or her number is: _____

❑ Get in contact with other effective people who can help (e.g., friends or family, people from group). These people include (with contact information):

_____

_____

❑ Get rid of the temptations (e.g., drugs, comfort food); surround myself with cues for effective behaviors (e.g., workout clothes, fruit).

❑ Review skills and handouts from DBT. The most helpful skills/handouts for me are:

_____

_____

❑ Opposite action (Emotion Regulation Handout 10) can be rehearsed to fight guilt and shame. If no other option works, go to an anonymous meeting of any sort and publicly report your lapse.

❑ Building mastery and coping ahead for emotional situations (Emotion Regulation Handout 19), and checking the facts (Emotion Regulation Handout 8), can be used to fight feelings of being out of control.

(*continued on next page*)

❑ Interpersonal skills (Interpersonal Effectiveness Handouts 5–7), such as asking for help from family, friends, sponsors, ministers, or counselors, can also be helpful. If you are isolated, help can often be found via online support groups. These people or groups include:

_____

_____

❑ Conduct a chain analysis to analyze what prompted the lapse (General Handouts 7, 7a).

❑ Problem-solve right away to find a way to "get back on the wagon" and repair any damage you have done (Emotion Regulation Handout 12).

❑ Distract yourself, self-soothe, and improve the moment.

❑ Cheerlead myself (e.g., "One slip is not a disaster," "Don't give up," "Don't get willful," "I can still climb back on the wagon.") My cheerleading statements will include:

_____

_____

❑ Do pros and cons of stopping again *now*.

❑ Stay away from extreme thinking. Always look for the middle ground. Don't let one slip turn into a disaster. (Check each extreme thought I am giving up and the middle ground I am accepting.)

Extreme thinking:	Middle ground:
❑ I have not quit yet; therefore I am doomed and might as well give up.	❑ Relapsing once does not doom me to never stopping.
❑ Now that I've relapsed, I might as well keep going.	❑ I relapsed, but that does not mean I have to stay relapsed. I can be effective and get up now.
❑ I missed an appointment, so I'm done with treatment.	❑ I missed an appointment, but I can get in to see my therapist ASAP.
❑ Other:	❑ Other:
❑ Other:	❑ Other:

❑ Recommit to 100% total abstinence.

From Clean Mind to Clear Mind

Due Date: _____ Name: _____ Week Starting: _____

Check off each **clean mind** behavior you plan on changing this week. During the week, write down the **clear mind** behavior you did to replace **clean mind**.

CLEAN MIND BEHAVIORS	CLEAR MIND BEHAVIORS AS REPLACEMENTS
☐ **1.** Engaging in **apparently irrelevant** behaviors that in the past inevitably led to problem behavior.	_____
☐ **2.** Thinking, "I've learned my lesson."	_____
☐ **3. Believing, "I can control my addiction."**	_____
☐ **4. Thinking, "I don't really have an addiction."**	_____
☐ **5.** Stopping or cutting back medication that helps with addiction.	_____
☐ **6.** Being in addiction environments.	_____
☐ **7.** Seeing friends who are still addicted.	_____
☐ **8.** Living with people who are addicted.	_____
☐ **9.** Keeping addiction paraphernalia.	_____
☐ **10.** Carrying around extra money.	_____
☐ **11.** Being irresponsible with bills.	_____
☐ **12.** Dressing like an addict.	_____
☐ **13.** Not going to meetings.	_____
☐ **14.** Isolating.	_____
☐ **15.** Believing, "I can do this alone."	_____
☐ **16.** Ignoring problems fueling addiction.	_____
☐ **17.** Acting as if I only need willpower.	_____
☐ **18.** Thinking, "I don't need to say anything about my addiction."	_____
☐ **19.** Thinking, "I can't stand this!"	_____
☐ **20.** Other: _____	_____
☐ **21.** Other: _____	_____

Reinforcing Nonaddictive Behaviors

Due Date: _____ Name: _____ Week Starting: _____

Check off and describe each effort you made to replace **addiction reinforcers** with **abstinence reinforcers.**

❏ 1. Searched for people to spend time with who aren't addicted. Describe what you did and who you found.

_____

_____

❏ 2. Increased number of enjoyable, nonaddictive activities. Describe activities.

_____

_____

❏ 3. Sampled different groups and different activities. Describe what you did and what you found.

_____

_____

❏ 4. Took one or more action steps to build positive events to replace addiction. Describe.

_____

_____

Check off and describe your **abstinence-sampling** efforts.

❏ 5. Committed to _____ days of abstinence. (Stayed abstinent _____ days.)

Describe abstinence plan and how you implemented it. *(See Distress Tolerance Worksheet 14.)*

❏ 6. Observe and describe positive events that occurred when you were *not* engaging in addictive behaviors.

Nonaddictive activity	**Positive events and consequences**
_____	_____
_____	_____
_____	_____

Burning Bridges and Building New Ones

Due Date: _____ Name: _____ Week Starting: _____

Rate the strength of your slamming the door on your addiction, from 0 (no intention of quitting addictive behavior) to 100 (complete and absolute commitment): _____. Go into Wise Mind and rate your level of slamming the door again: _____.

List all the things in your life that make addiction possible. Check those you get rid of.

- ❑ _____
- ❑ _____
- ❑ _____

- ❑ _____
- ❑ _____
- ❑ _____

List *all* tempting people, websites, and other contact information you need to continue addictive behaviors. Check those you erase or otherwise get rid of.

- ❑ _____
- ❑ _____
- ❑ _____

- ❑ _____
- ❑ _____
- ❑ _____

List all the things that would make addiction impossible. Check those that you do.

- ❑ _____
- ❑ _____
- ❑ _____

- ❑ _____
- ❑ _____
- ❑ _____

Describe imagery you can use to help reduce cravings:

Check and describe each strategy you have used to battle addiction urges.

❑ Kept new imagery in mind when urges hit: _____

_____

❑ Looked at moving images: _____

❑ Surrounded self with new smells: _____

❑ Urge-surfed: _____

Practicing Alternate Rebellion and Adaptive Denial

Due Date: _____ Name: _____ Week Starting: _____

Check and describe plans for alternate rebellion when the urge for addictive behaviors arises:

❑ 1. _____

❑ 2. _____

❑ 3. _____

Check and describe what you actually did as alternative behaviors instead of giving in to addictive behaviors:

❑ 1. _____

❑ 2. _____

Circle how effective alternate rebellion was at helping you survive the urges without giving in to addiction.

1	2	3	4	5
Not effective		Somewhat effective		Very effective

Check off and describe adaptive denial skills below that you used to manage urges:

❑ 1. Reframing an urge for a problem behavior as an urge for something else: _____
_____

Circle how effective this was at helping you survive the urges without giving in to addiction.

1	2	3	4	5
Not effective		Somewhat effective		Very effective

❑ 2. Putting off addictive behavior for ____ minutes, ____ times: _____
_____

Circle how effective this was at helping you survive the urges without giving in to addiction.

1	2	3	4	5
Not effective		Somewhat effective		Very effective

❑ 3. Reminded myself I only had to be abstinent for an hour, a day,
or _____.

_____

Circle how effective this was at helping you survive the urges without giving in to addiction.

1	2	3	4	5
Not effective		Somewhat effective		Very effective

Index